A USMLE STEP 1 REVIEW

Pharmacolo

*8*th Edition

A USMLE STEP 1 REVIEW

Pharmacology

8TH EDITION

700

Questions and Answers

Joseph J. Krzanowski, Jr., PhD
Professor and Vice Chair, Department of Pharmacology
University of South Florida, College of Medicine
Tampa, Florida

James B. Polson, PhD
Professor
Department of Pharmacology & Therapeutics
University of South Florida, College of Medicine
Tampa, Florida

Robert A. Woodbury, MD, PhD
Professor Emeritus of Pharmacology
Graduate School of Medical Science, University of Tennessee
Memphis, Tennessee

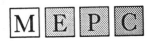

APPLETON & LANGE
Stamford, Connecticut

Copyright © 1996 by Appleton & Lange
A Simon & Schuster Company
© 1991 by Elsevier Science Publishing Co., Inc.

96 97 98 99 / 10 9 8 7 6 5 4 3 2 1

Prentice Hall International (UK) Limited, *London*
Prentice Hall of Australia Pty. Limited, *Sydney*
Prentice Hall Canada. Inc., *Toronto*
Prentice Hall Hispanoamericana. S.A., *Mexico*
Prentice Hall of India Private Limited, *New Delhi*
Prentice Hall of Japan, Inc., *Tokyo*
Simon & Schuster Asia Pte. Ltd., *Singapore*
Editora Prentice Hall do Brasil Ltda., *Rio de Janeiro*
Prentice Hall, *Englewood Cliffs. New Jersey*

ISBN 0-8385-6227-2

9 780838 562277   90000

ISBN: 0-8385-6227-2
ISSN: 1081-8839

Acquisitions Editor: Marinita Timban
Production Service: Inkwell Publishing Services
Designer: Mary Skudlarek

PRINTED IN THE UNITED STATES OF AMERICA

Dedication
Robert A. Woodbury, MD, PhD

The eighth edition of this book is dedicated to a scientist and educator who always expected the best from students, staff, and colleagues. This year he celebrates his 90th birthday and he continues to seek and communicate knowledge. His outstanding contribution to science and education over many decades is an example for all young people as they endeavor to master the science of pharmacology.

Contents

Preface

This eighth edition of *Pharmacology* has been substantially revised and updated to include current expanding knowledge in pharmacology. It is designed to assist you in preparing for course examinations and the USMLE Step 1.

There are 700 questions from each important area of pharmacology, organized in broad categories to give you a representative sampling of the material covered in course work, while helping you to determine those general areas in which you require intensive review.

An explanatory answer, referenced to widely available text and reference books, is included for each question and follows each section. For each question, specific page references to more than one textbook are usually provided, as students may have one textbook and not another. The authors suggest that the student consult the Answers and Discussion section immediately after answering several questions so as to discard the incorrect portions of each question and retain the correct knowledge. This book should serve to test your memory and ability to read questions carefully. Do not compromise by simply noting the correct answer and reading the explanatory comments; use the questions to test for areas of weakness. Do not be discouraged if you fail to achieve a high test score, since one benefit from the book is determining where additional review is most needed.

The purpose of this book is to provide a general review of pharmacology. The authors wish to encourage you to consult your textbooks for more in-depth coverage of the subject matter.

Special Acknowledgment

The authors would like to thank Karen M. Krzanowski, PharmD, Staff Pharmacist, H. Lee Moffitt Cancer Hospital, Tampa, Florida.

1

Principles of Pharmacology

DIRECTIONS (Questions 1-58): Each of the questions or incomplete statements below is followed by five suggested answers or completions. Select the **one** that is best in each case.

1. Assume Figure 1 represents quantal dose-effect plots. If curve 1 represents the therapeutic effect and curve 2 a toxic effect, which of the following numbers best approximates the therapeutic index?
   A. 1.2
   B. 5.5
   C. 15.0
   D. 36.5
   E. 48.0

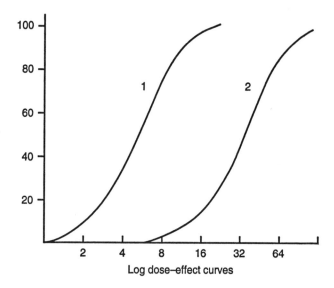

Figure 1 Log dose-effect curves.

2. All of the following statements are true EXCEPT
   A. the 1906 Pure Food and Drug Act prohibited the mislabeling and adulteration of drugs
   B. the birth defect, phocomelia, caused by thalidomide resulted in the passage in 1962 of the Kefauver-Harris Amendment to the Food, Drug, and Cosmetic Act requiring proof of safety by research on animals before a new drug may be tested in humans
   C. where there is no satisfactory treatment for a life-threatening disease, the Food and Drug Administration (FDA) may approve limited therapeutic use in humans of a new drug showing some efficacy and not unreasonable toxicity before data are presented for approval of general marketing of the new drug
   D. the 1984 Drug Price Competition and Patent Restriction Act allowed Abbreviated Drug Application (ADA) use for patented drugs to be sold under their generic name
   E. once a new drug application (NDA) is approved, other companies may apply to FDA to market this drug under the generic name

3. Which of the following statements is true?
   A. The rate of absorption and the rate of elimination of a drug are usually equal
   B. Plotted on an arithmetic scale, drug elimination follows a straight line
   C. A constant fraction of the drug in the body is eliminated per unit of time
   D. The elimination half-time of a drug is one half of the time required for the elimination of all of the drug
   E. None of the above

4. A drug dose repeated at the elimination half-life, just prior to the third administration, approaches the steady state of further administrations by what percentage?
   A. 50%
   B. 62.5%
   C. 75%
   D. 82.5%
   E. 90%

5. Different lots of a drug preparation have the same bioavailability when they
   A. are chemically equivalent
   B. fulfill the same chemical standards as set by regulatory agencies
   C. yield similar concentrations of the drug in blood and tissues
   D. have been approved by the Food and Drug Administration (FDA)
   E. meet the standards set forth by the United States Pharmacopeia (USP)

6. Passage of a drug through cell membranes is influenced by all of these factors EXCEPT
   A. its pH
   B. its type of action
   C. the amount of protein binding
   D. its lipid solubility
   E. the presence of pores in the membrane

7. Barriers to penetration of drugs into tissues vary in their effectiveness. Which of the following is the most effective barrier?
   A. Placenta early in pregnancy
   B. Placenta late in pregnancy
   C. Brain
   D. Tunica propria of testes
   E. Sertoli cells of testes

8. Passage of drugs across the cell membrane can be through solution in the membrane lipids and is governed by the permeability coefficient times the diffusion area times the concentration gradient. All the following statements are true concerning the passage of drugs EXCEPT
   A. for lipid-soluble (nonpolar) drugs the permeability coefficient is large
   B. for water-soluble (polar) drugs the permeability coefficient is small
   C. the rate of diffusion is independent of the surface area for transfer
   D. the passage of drugs is facilitated by a high concentration gradient
   E. the passage of drugs is facilitated across the lung because of its very large surface area

9. Which of the following statements is true?
   A. The protein-bound drug is the portion of drug that is therapeutically active
   B. Drugs cross the placenta mainly by active transport
   C. The LD_{50} is 50% of the minimum dose that is lethal to animals of a specified species and strain
   D. The LD_{50} is 50% of the average dose that is lethal to animals of a specific species or strain
   E. The maximal intensity of a specified therapeutic effect that a drug is able to produce is referred to as its efficacy

10. Which of the following factors modifies the movement of drug molecules from the site of administration into the body and bodily components?
   A. Lipid diffusion
   B. Aqueous diffusion
   C. Facilitative diffusion (special carriers)

D. Receptor-mediated endocytosis (pinocytosis)
E. All of the above

11. The signature of a prescription consists of
    A. the names and the amounts of each ingredient
    B. your signature and address
    C. your signature
    D. instructions for the patient as to how and when the medication is to be taken
    E. the quantity to be dispensed

12. Orphan drugs meet all of the following criteria EXCEPT
    A. for patients with rare genetic deficiencies
    B. for the treatment of rare diseases
    C. where the disease population is very young
    D. where the incidence of the disease is too large
    E. where proof of the drug safety must be established in small populations

13. All of the following statements about clinical trials of new drugs are true EXCEPT
    A. in phase 1, dose-dependent effects are studied in healthy volunteers
    B. in phase 2, effects are studied in a small number of patients who have been diagnosed with the target disease
    C. in phase 3, studies are often carried out in much larger populations than phase 1 and in clinical settings similar to the proposed use of the drug
    D. acute and subacute animal toxicity studies are completed before testing in humans
    E. it can be expected that toxic effects with a frequency of 1/10,000 will be detected in phase 3 clinical trials

14. In which formal phase of clinical trials are pharmacokinetic measurements made and drug metabolism studied?
    A. Phase 1
    B. Phase 2
    C. Phase 3
    D. Phase 4
    E. None of the above

15. On repeated use all of the following drugs may lead to enzyme induction of cytochrome P-450 EXCEPT
    A. isoniazid
    B. ethanol (chronic use)
    C. phenobarbital
    D. phenytoin
    E. digoxin

16. The most common cause(s) of slow acetylation of isoniazid is (are)
    A. genetic variations
    B. sex-dependent variations
    C. pulmonary disease
    D. diabetes
    E. hyperthyroidism

17. All of the following statements about drug-metabolizing enzymes are true EXCEPT
    A. phenylbutazone induces microsomal enzymes
    B. cimetidine inhibits the enzymatic biotransformation of warfarin
    C. phenobarbital inhibits the enzymatic biotransformation of warfarin
    D. secobarbital inhibits its own metabolism by cytochrome P-450
    E. hepatic microsomal oxidases are often markedly reduced by hepatic disease

18. Cardiac disease is likely to reduce the hepatic clearance of all of the following drugs EXCEPT
    A. propranolol
    B. phenobarbital
    C. verapamil
    D. morphine
    E. lidocaine

19. All of the following biotransformation reactions are classified as phase 2 EXCEPT
    A. glucuronidations
    B. acetylations
    C. reductions
    D. methylations
    E. glutathione conjugation

20. The Federal Food, Drug, and Cosmetic Act and its amendments contain all of the following legal provisions EXCEPT
   A. they vest the FDA with power to approve or disapprove the marketing of a drug
   B. they require new drugs to be safe
   C. they vest the FDA with power to regulate how a drug is used by physicians
   D. they establish guidelines for reporting information about adverse reactions, clinical testing, and advertising of new drugs
   E. they require proof of efficacy for new drugs

21. Which of the following drug-induced effects is (are) more likely to be discovered by vigilant postmarketing surveillance of a new drug than by phase 3 clinical trials?
   A. Effects in pregnant women
   B. Rare toxicities
   C. Efficacy for a particular indication that is unsuspected based on phase 1 and phase 2 data
   D. Effects in children
   E. All of the above

22. Hepatic drug metabolism is often decreased by all of the following disease states EXCEPT
   A. diseases affecting liver architecture or function
   B. heavy metal poisoning
   C. cardiac disease
   D. hyperthyroidism
   E. malignant hepatic tumors

23. Concerning potency and efficacy
   A. potency refers to the maximal effect a drug is capable of producing
   B. efficacy refers to lack of toxicity of a drug
   C. efficacy refers to the amount of a drug required to produce one-half of the maximal effect
   D. their efficacy is more important than their potency when comparing the usefulness of morphine and codeine as analgesics
   E. their potency is more important than their efficacy when comparing the usefulness of morphine and codeine as analgesics

24. Conditions responsible for excessive or unusual drug effects include
   A. unusual sensitivity, either allergic in nature or an idiosyncratic reaction
   B. administration of the drug too frequently or for a prolonged period of time
   C. the presence of other drugs
   D. the age of the individual
   E. all of the above

25. The rate of urinary excretion of acidic drugs such as aspirin and barbiturates is increased by
   A. administration of sodium bicarbonate
   B. administration of ammonium chloride
   C. administration of ascorbic acid
   D. keeping the urine at neutral pH
   E. none of the above

26. Ionized and/or lipid-insoluble drugs
   A. may pass through the small aqueous channels, or pores, of cells of many tissues
   B. generally do not gain entry to brain cells
   C. cross biologic lipid membranes less readily than do non-ionized drugs
   D. all of the above
   E. none of the above

27. Drug responsiveness to the same drug may vary in a single individual during treatment course or vary among individuals. Causes of this variation could include
   A. presence of other drugs
   B. very young or very old patients
   C. tolerance to the drug effect
   D. idiosyncratic response to the drug
   E. all of the above

28. Excretion of drugs via the kidney involves which of the following mechanisms?
   A. Passive glomerular filtration
   B. Active tubular excretion

C. Passive tubular reabsorption
D. All of the above
E. None of the above

29. Clinical trials evaluating new drugs require
   A. informed consent (where possible)
   B. adverse reactions to the new drug to be immediately reported to the FDA
   C. use of placebo (where possible)
   D. use of a standard control drug for comparison (where possible)
   E. all of the above

30. All of the following statements about the blood-brain barrier are true EXCEPT
   A. it is poorly penetrated by water-soluble drugs
   B. it consists of glial cells surrounding the capillaries
   C. it is easily penetrated by ether
   D. it is penetrated more readily in patients with meningitis
   E. it is easily penetrated by penicillin under normal conditions

31. If a drug is a weak base so that some molecules are ionized and some are nonionized, which form will most readily diffuse across cell membranes by solution in the lipids?
   A. They both diffuse at the same rate
   B. The ionized molecules diffuse faster than the nonionized
   C. The nonionized molecules diffuse better than the ionized
   D. It depends on the particular drug
   E. It depends on the type of cell

32. Which of the following equations can be used to calculate the degree of ionization of weak acids, such as phenobarbital, in solution?
   A. The Fick equation
   B. The Michaelis-Menten equation
   C. The equation for first-order processes
   D. The equation for zero-order processes
   E. The Henderson-Hasselbalch equation

33. Which of the following mechanisms is most likely to cause **heterologous** desensitization of receptors?
    A. Feedback inactivation of an enzyme that is activated by several types of receptors
    B. Increased down-regulation, by endocytosis, of receptors for the agonist causing the desensitization
    C. Increased destruction of receptors for the agonist causing the desensitization
    D. Decreased synthesis of receptors for the agonist causing the desensitization
    E. Increased rate of recycling of receptors for the agonist causing the desensitization

34. The following statements refer to the binding of drugs to their specific receptors. All the statements are true EXCEPT
    A. agonist binding is usually reversible
    B. agonists cannot activate receptors without binding to them
    C. binding specificity often distinguishes between stereoisomers of the same molecule
    D. agonists activate receptors because they bind with greater affinity than antagonists
    E. agonist binding can be affected by other ligands binding at allosteric sites

35. Many drugs produce effects by interaction with receptors for endogenous hormones, neurotransmitters, cytokines, etc. Other cellular components with which drugs interact to produce effects include
    A. nucleic acids
    B. structural proteins
    C. enzymes
    D. proteins involved in transport processes
    E. all of the above

36. Which of the following chemical compounds produce their major effects by binding to intracellular receptors that bind to nuclear DNA to regulate gene expression?
    A. Insulin
    B. Succinylcholine
    C. Catecholamines
    D. Opioid peptides
    E. Steroids

37. Which of the following statements best describes the "first pass effect"?

A. Orally administered drugs that are rapidly inactivated by hepatic enzymes or rapidly excreted in the bile lose much of their effectiveness on their first pass through the liver

B. Drugs actively secreted into the urine are almost completely cleared on their first pass through the kidneys

C. The first drug to pass into the circulation from the intestine is the first to produce its effect

D. A high initial concentration of drug passes through the circulation when intravenous bolus injection is used

E. Upon administration, drugs pass into well-perfused tissues before being redistributed to tissues that are less well perfused

38. Which of the following statements related to the binding of drugs by plasma proteins is true?

A. Bound drug is unable to diffuse into tissues until it becomes unbound

B. A drug that is bound by plasma proteins will have a smaller apparent volume of distribution than if it were not bound

C. Displacement of the bound drug by another drug can increase the effects of a given dosage of the first drug

D. Acidic drugs are bound mostly to plasma albumin

E. All of the above

39. Which of the following is LEAST likely to affect renal drug excretion?

A. Concomitant excretion of two drugs, both of which are weak acids

B. Concomitant excretion of two drugs, one a weak acid, the other a weak base

C. A decrease in glomerular filtration rate

D. Displacement of a drug from plasma protein binding sites

E. An increase in renal blood flow

40. Which of the following would be the likely result of a decrease in urinary pH?

A. Decreased urinary excretion of a weak base

B. Increased urinary excretion of a weak acid

C. Increased urinary excretion of a weak base

D. Decreased urinary excretion of a nonionized drug

E. Increased urinary excretion of a completely ionized drug

41. All of the following are assumptions of Classical Occupancy Theory (Clark and Ariens) EXCEPT
   A. the interaction between drugs and receptors are simple bimolecular reactions
   B. the interaction between drugs and receptors follows the Law of Mass Action
   C. the effect caused by a drug is proportional to the number of receptors it occupies
   D. the maximal effect of a drug is achieved when only a fraction of the receptors are occupied
   E. one-half of the maximal effect is achieved when half of the receptors are occupied

42. All of the following statements about partial agonists are true EXCEPT
   A. they can reduce the effects of full agonists acting at the same receptor sites
   B. even at high concentrations, they are unable to occupy 100% of the receptors
   C. even at high concentrations, they are unable to elicit responses as large as those elicited by full agonists
   D. their effects can be blocked by noncompetitive antagonists
   E. their effects can be blocked by competitive antagonists

43. The term that refers to the rapid diminution of responsiveness following administration of a drug is
   A. hyporeactivity
   B. idiosyncratic drug response
   C. tolerance
   D. drug inactivation
   E. tachyphylaxis

44. Which of the following factors can cause variations from patient to patient in response to drugs that act on endogenous ligand receptors?
   A. Variation in the concentration of drug that reaches the receptor
   B. Variation in the concentration of the endogenous ligand that activates the receptor
   C. Variation in the number or function of receptors
   D. Variation in components of the response mechanism distal to the receptor
   E. All of the above

45. Which of the following mechanisms is common to the synaptic transmitters: acetylcholine, Gamma-aminobutyric acid, glycine, aspartate and glutamate?
  A. They regulate the flow of ions through plasma membrane channels
  B. They activate tyrosine kinases through transmembrane receptors
  C. They activate G_s-guanine nucleotide binding proteins
  D. They bind to receptors that regulate gene expression in the nucleus
  E. They activate soluble guanylyl cyclase

46. Which of the following enzymes is activated as a result of the interaction of catecholamines with α_1-adrenergic receptors?
  A. Adenylyl cyclase
  B. Cyclic GMP phosphodiesterase
  C. Tyrosine kinase
  D. Phospholipase C
  E. Guanylyl cyclase

47. What is the mechanism of action of drugs that activate β-adrenergic receptors?
  A. They increase intracellular levels of phosphoinositides
  B. They activate adenylyl cyclase, causing an increase in cyclic AMP formation
  C. They open agonist-responsive Ca^{2+} channels
  D. They open K^+ channels causing hyperpolarization of cell membranes
  E. They activate G_i-guanine nucleotide-binding proteins to attenuate adenylyl cyclase activity

48. Which of the following effects are common among drugs that activate the following receptor subtypes: a_2-adrenergic, muscarinic acetylcholine, D_1-dopaminergic, S_1-serotonergic?
  A. Opening of transmembrane Na^+ channels
  B. Increased rate of formation of cyclic AMP by adenylyl cyclase
  C. Attenuation of adenylyl cyclase activation by agonists
  D. Activation of cyclic GMP phosphodiesterase
  E. Activation of membrane bound guanylyl cyclase

49. The hypothesis that the pharmacological or toxic effects of a drug in the body are related to the drug concentration in the general circulation is true
   A. for all drugs
   B. for many drugs
   C. only for drugs that penetrate the "blood-brain barrier"
   D. only for antibiotics
   E. for no drugs

50. All of the following statements about the Volume of Distribution (V_d) of drugs in the body are true EXCEPT
   A. it relates the blood or plasma concentration to the amount of drug in the body
   B. it is the volume throughout which the drug is distributed in the body
   C. it can change in an individual with age
   D. it can change due to disease
   E. none of the above

51. Which of the following factors affect the bioavailability of an orally administered drug?
   A. The fraction absorbed from the intestine
   B. Metabolism of the drug in the intestine and/or intestinal wall
   C. Metabolism of the drug in the portal blood and/or liver
   D. Biliary excretion of the drug
   E. All of the above

52. Which of the following statements about drug clearance is true?
   A. Steady state plasma concentrations are determined mainly by the relationship between total clearance and dosing rate
   B. Plasma clearance by the kidneys equals the renal rate of elimination divided by plasma concentration
   C. Clearance may be defined based on drug concentration in the blood or plasma, or on the concentration of unbound drug in the circulation
   D. The total systemic clearance is the sum of hepatic clearance + renal clearance + clearance by other organs
   E. All of the above

53. Which of the following statements about drug elimination is NOT true?
   A. For most drugs, elimination follows first-order kinetics
   B. For most drugs, a constant fraction of the drug is eliminated per unit of time
   C. The hepatic rate of elimination is the amount of drug entering minus the amount exiting the liver per unit of time
   D. For most drugs, the mechanisms for elimination are saturated by therapeutic plasma concentrations
   E. None of the above

54. What would be the half-life of a drug with a distribution of 0.15 L/kg and a clearance of 48 mL/min in a 70-kg man?
   A. 1.5 hr
   B. 2.5 hr
   C. 4.5 hr
   D. 8.5 hr
   E. 24 hr

55. What rate of intravenous infusion is needed to maintain theophylline plasma levels at 15 µg/mL in a 70-kg man? The systemic clearance of theophylline is 48 mL/min
   A. 130 µg/min
   B. 235 µg/min
   C. 340 µg/min
   D. 550 µg/min
   E. 720 µg/min

56. What orally administered loading dose would achieve a plasma concentration of 10 µg/mL for a drug that has a volume of distribution (V_d) of 100 L and 75% bioavailability?
   A. 1.3 mg
   B. 3.6 mg
   C. 12 mg
   D. 24 mg
   E. 48 mg

57. All of the following statements are true EXCEPT

- **A.** biotransformation of drugs in the body usually yields products that diffuse across renal tubular membranes less readily than the parent compounds
- **B.** biotransformation reactions often yield products that are inactive pharmacologically
- **C.** biotransformation reactions can yield products that are pharmacologically more active than the parent compound
- **D.** biotransformation reactions usually yield products that are more lipophilic than the parent compound
- **E.** in some cases, biotransformation reactions enhance the toxicity of chemicals introduced into the body

58. Which of the following are characteristic of phase 2 biotransformation reactions?

- **A.** They oxidase primary amines
- **B.** They hydroxylate aliphatic compounds
- **C.** They conjugate compounds with endogenous substances such as glucuronic acid or sulfate
- **D.** They hydrolyze esters
- **E.** They reduce carbonyl oxygen to form hydroxyl groups

DIRECTIONS (Questions 59–70): The group of questions below consists of five lettered headings followed by a list of numbered words or phrases. For each numbered word or phrase, select the one lettered heading that is most closely associated with it. Each lettered heading may be selected once, more than once, or not at all.

Questions 59–65: Drug action is reduced mainly by

- **A.** oxidation
- **B.** reduction
- **C.** hydrolysis
- **D.** conjugation
- **E.** excretion unchanged by the kidneys

59. Morphine

60. Phenobarbital

61. Digoxin

62. Theophylline

63. Procaine

64. Acetaminophen

65. Ethanol

Questions 66–70: The levels of enzymes involved in drug metabolism are under genetic influence. Match the defect-drug with the clinical consequences

    A. INI-acetylation defect; isoniazid
    B. Ester hydrolysis defect: tolbutamide
    C. Hydroxylation defect: warfarin
    D. Oxidation defect: debrisoquin (antihypertensive)
    E. Pseudocholinesterase defect: succinylcholine

66. Cardiotoxicity

67. Bleeding

68. Peripheral neuropathy

69. Prolonged apnea

70. Orthostatic hypotension

Principles of Pharmacology

Answers and Discussion

1. **B.** The therapeutic index is $LD_{50}/ED_{50} = 32/5.8 = 5.5$. (**Ref. 1,** pp. 29–30; **Ref. 4,** pp. 67–69; **Ref. 12,** pp. 27–28)

2. **E.** The 1906 Pure Food and Drug Act has been modified to add new goals and to solve new problems. The many amendments were added to protect the public. Because of the great expense involved in developing a new drug that meets the FDA rules and regulations, the new drug is the property of the company that developed it. However, to make some drugs less expensive, the 1984 Drug Price Competition and Patent Term Restoration Act was passed. This Act allows certain older drugs to be marketed by other companies without proving efficacy again. Bioequivalence must be established. In exchange, patent life can be extended under restrictive conditions. (**Ref. 1,** pp. 64–67; **Ref. 4,** pp. 74–75; **Ref. 12,** pp. 66–68)

3. **C.** Drug elimination follows an exponential decay curve when plotted on an arithmetic scale. Elimination half-life is the time required for one half of the drug to be eliminated. It takes several elimination half-times for the body to rid itself of all of the drug. (**Ref. 1,** pp. 38–40; **Ref. 4,** pp. 23–25; **Ref. 12,** pp. 34–38)

4. **C.** With two doses, 75% of the plateau blood level will be reached. With antibiotics and a few other drugs, the first dose is

frequently doubled so that the plateau (steady state) is approached with the first dose. (**Ref. 1,** pp. 42–45; **Ref. 4,** pp. 23–30; **Ref. 12,** pp. 42–44)

5. **C.** Several preparations may be composed of the same chemicals and meet regulatory chemical standards but differ in particle size or crystalline form so that rate and amount of absorption differ. Consequently, they would not possess the same bioavailability. (**Ref. 1,** pp. 41–42; **Ref. 4,** p. 26; **Ref. 12,** pp. 39–40)

6. **B.** All of the factors listed, except the type of action of a drug, influence the passage of drugs through cell membranes; however, highly lipid-soluble drugs can enter the central nervous system (CNS) even though pores are not present. Aqueous-soluble drugs encounter a barrier in the absence of pores. (**Ref. 1,** pp. 2–4; **Ref. 4,** pp. 3–5; **Ref. 12,** pp. 4–6)

7. **E.** Sertoli cells of the testes are tightly packed together, forming an effective barrier to drug penetration. (**Ref. 2,** p. 32)

8. **C.** In Fick's law of diffusion: flux = permeability coefficient × diffusion area × concentration gradient. The coefficient for a non-polar drug is large and for polar drugs is small. A high concentration gradient and a large surface area would facilitate the passage of drugs across a membrane or tissue. (**Ref. 1,** p. 4; **Ref. 12,** p. 5)

9. **E.** Only an unbound drug is therapeutically active. Drugs readily diffuse across the placenta. The LD_{50} is the dose that is lethal to 50% of the animals. Efficacy refers to the potential maximal therapeutic effect. (**Ref. 1,** pp. 28–30; **Ref. 4,** p. 67; **Ref. 12,** pp. 27–28)

10. **E.** The diffusion, or movement process, is dependent on a number of factors including lipid and water solubility, facilitative diffusion, and pinocytosis. (**Ref. 1,** pp. 2–4; **Ref. 4,** p. 4; **Ref. 9,** p. 23; **Ref. 12,** pp. 4–5)

11. **D.** In a prescription, the signature is the instructions for the patient; the name and amount of each ingredient is known as the inscription; the quantity to be dispensed is known as the subscription. (**Ref. 1,** pp. 915–916; **Ref. 4,** pp. 1641–1643; **Ref. 9,** p. 108; **Ref. 12,** pp. 970–972)

12. D. Under normal FDA-NDA rules drugs designed to benefit a small segment of a population would be far more expensive to market than the income generated by the sales to such a small market. The Orphan Drug Act was designed to help industry develop these drugs for the limited market. (**Ref. 1,** pp. 66–67; **Ref. 4,** pp. 74–78; **Ref. 12,** p. 68)

13. E. In order to detect toxic effects with a frequency of 1/10,000, 180,000 subjects must be exposed. Toxicities of this frequency are more likely to be found in postmarket surveillance programs than in premarketing clinical testing phases. (**Ref. 1,** pp. 65–66; **Ref. 4,** pp. 75–77; **Ref. 12,** pp. 67–68)

14. A. In phase 1, initial studies are made on the biological effects, safety, pharmacokinetics, and metabolism in humans. (**Ref. 1,** p. 65; **Ref. 4,** pp. 75–77; **Ref. 12,** p. 67)

15. E. Induced cytochrome P-450 activity may increase the metabolism of the drug that stimulated the enzyme activity. Isoniazid, ethanol used chronically, phenobarbital, and phenytoin are some of the main drugs that induce cytochrome P-450 activity. (**Ref. 1,** pp. 51–52, 57–58; **Ref. 4,** pp. 17–18; **Ref. 12,** pp. 51–53)

16. A. Genetic polymorphism accounts for a slow acetylation phenotype in about 50% of the U.S. population. The polymorphism is race-dependent worldwide. (**Ref. 1,** p. 56; **Ref. 4,** pp. 1147–1148; **Ref. 12,** pp. 55–56)

17. C. Phenobarbital accelerates biotransformation of warfarin by induction of hepatic cytochrome P-450. (**Ref. 1,** p. 58; **Ref. 4,** pp. 71, 1320; **Ref. 12,** p. 57)

18. B. Cardiac disease impairs elimination of drugs that are cleared by the liver at very high rates. The overall rate of hepatic metabolism is therefore dependent on blood flow through the liver. Of the drugs listed, the metabolism of all except phenobarbital is flow-limited. (**Ref. 1,** p. 59; **Ref. 4,** pp. 17, 22–23; **Ref. 12,** p. 58)

19. C. Conjugation reactions are classified as phase 2. Reductions do not involve conjugation of the drug with an endogenous molecule or radical. (**Ref. 1,** pp. 53–55; **Ref. 4,** pp. 15–17; **Ref. 12,** pp. 52–53)

20. C. The FDA can approve or disapprove a drug for general use but it cannot regulate how a drug is used. Such regulation would interfere with the practice of medicine. (**Ref. 4,** p. 75)

21. E. After a drug is released for marketing, populations that are almost never studied in premarketing trials are exposed to it, including pregnant women, children, and patients with concomitant diseases. The much greater number of subjects makes it possible to detect rare effects that may not be found in the smaller number of patients studied in phase 3 trials. (**Ref. 1,** p. 67; **Ref. 4,** p. 77; **Ref. 12,** pp. 64–65)

22. D. Hyperthyroidism does not decrease hepatic metabolism, but it does increase the metabolism of antipyrine, digoxin, methimazole, and practolol. Acute or chronic liver diseases impair hepatic metabolism. Cardiac disease impairs elimination of those drugs whose rate of metabolism is limited by hepatic blood flow. (**Ref. 1,** pp. 58–59; **Ref. 12,** p. 58)

23. D. Confusion between potency and efficacy sometimes occurs. Potency is determined by finding the dose required to produce a given effect. Comparison of drug potency is relatively unimportant unless the ratio for doses is different for potency and toxic effects. Comparison of drugs for efficacy is important because efficacy refers to the maximal therapeutic effect that can be obtained. In severe pain, codeine is ineffective, even with increased doses. (**Ref. 1,** pp. 28–29; **Ref. 4,** p. 67; **Ref. 12,** pp. 27–28)

24. E. These are only a few of the conditions that modify drug effects. Administration of a drug for a prolonged period can cause increased effects due to accumulation of the drug or due to cumulative effects without any increased drug levels, or it may cause decreased actions due to tolerance. Infants and elderly patients are more sensitive to many drugs, particularly those that depress the central nervous system. (**Ref. 1,** pp. 45–47, 56–59; **Ref. 4,** pp. 17–18; **Ref. 12,** pp. 55–57)

25. A. Sodium bicarbonate causes the urine to become alkaline, thereby reducing reabsorption of acidic drugs by the tubules. Excretion, therefore, is increased. (**Ref. 1,** p. 2; **Ref. 4,** pp. 4–5; **Ref. 12,** pp. 5–6)

26. D. Ionized and/or lipid-insoluble drugs do reach most cells by passage through pores; however, this is not the case for brain cells because of the blood-brain barrier. (**Ref. 1,** pp. 2–3; **Ref. 4,** pp. 4–5; **Ref. 12,** p. 4)

27. E. The variation of drug response during a single course of therapy and variations among individuals are due to many factors including drug interactions, age, sex, pregnancy, weight, and unexpected sensitivity and responses. (**Ref. 1,** pp. 45–47, 56–59; **Ref. 4,** pp. 17–18, 30; **Ref. 12,** pp. 55–57)

28. D. When a drug is excreted by the kidneys, one or more of the following are responsible: glomerular filtration, active tubular secretion, and passive tubular reabsorption. (**Ref. 1,** p. 6; **Ref. 4,** pp. 18–20; **Ref. 12,** p. 38)

29. E. The FDA requires informed patient consent, reports of adverse effects and, where possible, the use of a placebo and a standard control drug for comparison to make the study more valid. (**Ref. 1,** pp. 63–67; **Ref. 4,** pp. 74–78; **Ref. 12,** pp. 65–66)

30. E. Penicillin does not penetrate the blood-brain barrier under normal conditions; however, the inflammation present in meningitis modifies its permeability, permitting the penetration by penicillin. (**Ref. 1,** p. 629; **Ref. 4,** p. 11; **Ref. 12,** p. 683)

31. C. Ionized drugs are lipid-insoluble whereas nonionized forms are lipid soluble and can dissolve in and diffuse across lipid cell membranes. (**Ref. 1,** p. 2; **Ref. 4,** p. 4; **Ref. 12,** pp. 5–6)

32. E. For weak acids, ionization can be represented by: HA $\rightleftharpoons$ $H^+ + A^-$. The Henderson-Hasselbalch equation calculates the degree of ionization as $\log(HA/A^-) = pKa - pH$, where pKa is the $-\log$ (equilibrium dissociation constant for the weak acid) and the pH is the pH of the environment. Ionization of weak bases can be represented by: $H^+ + B \rightleftharpoons HB^+$, and the corresponding form of the Henderson-Hasselbalch equation is $\log (HB^+/B) = pKa - pH$. (**Ref. 1,** pp. 2–4; **Ref. 4,** pp. 4–5; **Ref. 12,** p. 5)

33. A. Heterologous desensitization refers to a decreased effectiveness of drugs acting through different classes of receptors after exposure of cells to a single pharmacological agonist. This can be caused by modification of each class of receptors by a common feedback mechanism, or by effects at some common point in the effector pathway. (**Ref. 4**, p. 40)

34. D. The ability of a drug to activate its receptor *(intrinsic activity)* is believed to depend on its ability to induce conformational changes in the receptor, and is not dependent on its affinity. In fact, some antagonists bind receptors with higher affinities than agonists. Agonist binding is usually reversible, often distinguishes between subtle molecular differences such as stereoisomerism, and can be affected by other ligands that bind to allosteric sites. (**Ref. 1**, pp. 10–11, 14–15; **Ref. 4**, pp. 33–34, 43–44; **Ref. 12**, p. 9)

35. E. Examples of drugs can be found that produce effects as the result of their interaction with nucleic acids (dactinomycin), structural proteins (colchicine), enzymes (methotrexate), and transport proteins (digitalis glycosides). (**Ref. 1**, pp. 10–11; **Ref. 4**, pp. 675, 817, 1224, 1241; **Ref. 12**, pp. 9–10)

36. E. Steroid hormones and drugs that interact with steroid receptors produce effects by activating cytosolic receptors, which bind to nuclear DNA and regulate the expression of specific genes. Succinylcholine binds to and opens ion channels at the neuromuscular junction. Insulin produces its effects by binding to receptors that activate intracellular tyrosine kinases. Catecholamines and opioid peptides bind to receptors that are coupled to guanine-binding proteins (G-proteins) that regulate enzymes and/or ion channels. (**Ref. 1**, pp. 17–24; **Ref. 4**, pp. 35–40, 171, 488, 489; **Ref. 12**, pp. 17–26)

37. A. The "first pass effect" refers to the decrease in bioavailability of an orally administered drug due to its elimination upon passage through the liver from the stomach or intestine. (**Ref. 1**, p. 42; **Ref. 4**, p. 5; **Ref. 12**, p. 49)

38. E. Because plasma proteins are generally confined to the circulation, protein-bound drugs cannot diffuse into tissues. The apparent volume of distribution is calculated using the plasma concentration (free plus bound drug) as one factor. Because bound drug is included in the plasma concentration, binding will decrease the calculated volume of distribution. Displacement of a drug from proteins may increase the concentration of free drug. Acidic drugs are bound mostly by albumin, whereas basic drugs are bound mostly by α_1-acid glycoprotein. (**Ref. 1,** pp. 38–39; **Ref. 4,** p. 1112; **Ref. 12,** p. 45)

39. **B.** A weak acid and weak base would not be expected to interfere with each other's excretion. Weak acids are usually excreted by saturable mechanisms in the proximal convoluted tubule, and two weak acids may compete with each other for this mechanism. Changes in glomerular flow rate, renal blood flow, or plasma protein binding will change the amount of drug filtered by the kidneys. (**Ref. 1,** p. 6; **Ref. 4,** pp. 18–20; **Ref. 12,** p. 38)

40. **C.** A decrease in urinary pH would increase the ionized and decrease the nonionized form of a weak base. Nonionized drug is reabsorbed, but ionized drug is trapped in the urine and excreted. Decreased urinary pH would decrease the ionized form of weak acids. (**Ref. 1,** p. 3; **Ref. 4,** pp. 18–29; **Ref. 12,** pp. 5–6)

41. **D.** Classical Occupancy Theory assumes that the maximal effect is achieved when all of the receptors are occupied. The possibility that maximal effect may be produced when only a fraction of the receptors are occupied was Stephenson's modification, often called the concept of "Spare Receptors." (**Ref. 1,** pp. 10–16; **Ref. 4,** pp. 43–47; **Ref. 12,** pp. 9–17)

42. **B.** Partial agonists combine with receptors to produce an effect, but they do not elicit effects as large as full agonists even at concentrations high enough to occupy 100% of the receptors. In Classical Occupancy Theory, the smaller efficacy of partial agonists is ascribed to smaller intrinsic activities. (**Ref. 1,** pp. 13–15; **Ref. 4,** pp. 46–47; **Ref. 12,** pp. 15–17)

43. **E.** Tachyphylaxis refers to a rapidly diminished responsiveness whereas tolerance refers to diminished responsiveness as a consequence of continued administration. Idiosyncratic responses are responses that are infrequent. Drug inactivation usually refers to biotransformation of a drug to inactive products, and hyporeactivity does not refer to a change in responsiveness but to a smaller than usual response in a given individual. (**Ref. 1,** p. 31; **Ref. 4,** pp. 67–68; **Ref. 12,** p. 29)

44. E. Patients may differ in rate of drug absorption, distribution, elimination (pharmacokinetics), concentration of the endogenous receptor ligand, number or function of receptors, or postreceptor mechanisms. All of these factors contribute to drug responsiveness in an individual. (**Ref. 1,** pp. 4–8, 28–32; **Ref. 4,** pp. 65–69; **Ref. 12,** pp. 29–30)

45. A. The nicotinic acetylcholine receptor and receptors for GABA, and excitatory aminoacids all open ion channels to increase transmembrane conductance of ions, thereby altering the electrical potential across cell membranes. (**Ref. 1,** pp. 18–22; **Ref. 4,** pp. 35–38; **Ref. 12,** p. 20)

46. D. Activation of α_1-adrenoceptors results in activation of a phosphoinositide-specific phospholipase C, which hydrolyzes phosphatidylinositol-4,5-bisphosphate to diacylglycerol (DAG) and inositol-1,4,5-triphosphate (IP_3). Both DAG and IP_3 are second messengers. DAG activates protein kinase C, causing the phosphorylation of protein substrates, and IP_3 releases Ca^{2+} from intracellular storage vesicles. (**Ref. 1,** pp. 22–27; **Ref. 7,** pp. 144–154)

47. B. Activation of β-adrenergic receptors activates G_s-guanine nucleotide-binding proteins, which activate adenylyl cyclase. The resulting accumulation of intracellular cyclic AMP causes activation of cyclic AMP-dependent protein kinase, which phosphorylates protein substrates. (**Ref. 1,** pp. 17–18; **Ref. 4,** pp. 35–40; **Ref. 12,** pp. 17–18)

48. C. Activation of α_2-adrenergic, muscarinic cholinergic, D_1-dopaminergic and S_1-serotonergic receptors activate G_i-guanine nucleotide binding proteins which attenuate the activation of adenylyl cyclase by drugs, hormones and neurotransmitters. (**Ref. 1,** pp. 22–26; **Ref. 12,** pp. 20–23)

49. B. For most drugs, the concentration in the general circulation is related to the concentration at the site of action. However, for some drugs, no clear relationship has been found between plasma concentrations and pharmacological effects. (**Ref. 1,** pp. 35, 38; **Ref. 4,** p. 20; **Ref. 12,** p. 33)

50. B. The V_d equals the amount of drug in body/blood or plasma concentration. It represents the volume throughout which a drug would be uniformly distributed to provide the blood or plasma concentration measured. However, due to drug binding to plasma and tissue proteins and distribution into fatty tissues, the V_d calculated by the equation may not represent the actual volume occupied by the drug. For example, the V_d for digoxin in a 70 kg man is about 645 liters. (**Ref. 1,** pp. 5–6; **Ref. 4,** pp. 23–25)

51. E. Bioavailability is usually defined as the *fraction* of unchanged drug that reaches the systemic circulation or its site of action after administration. In this case, the bioavailability of an intravenously administered drug is one. Bioavailability is alternatively defined as the *rate* at which the drug reaches the systemic circulation or site of action. For an orally administered dose, the absorption, biotransformation, or excretion of the drug prior to its reaching the systemic circulation or site of action all affect the drug's bioavailability. (**Ref. 1,** pp. 40–41; **Ref. 4,** p. 5)

52. E. Plasma concentrations reach a steady state when the dosage rate multiplied by the bioavailable fraction equals clearance. Plasma clearance (volume per unit of time) equals the rate of elimination of the drug divided by the plasma concentration. Alternative definitions may substitute blood or unbound drug concentrations for plasma concentrations in this formula. Total systemic clearance is the sum of the clearances by all organ systems. (**Ref. 1,** pp. 38–40; **Ref. 4,** pp. 21–23)

53. D. For most drugs, a constant *fraction* of the drug is eliminated per unit of time (first-order kinetics). In the unusual situation in which the mechanisms for elimination become saturated, a constant *amount* of drug is eliminated per unit of time (zero-order kinetics). The rate of elimination by an organ is calculated by the formula: $RE = Q\,C_A - Q\,C_v$, where Q is the blood flow through the organ, and C_A and C_v are arterial and venous drug concentrations, respectively. (**Ref. 1,** pp. 38–40; **Ref. 4,** pp. 21–23; **Ref. 12,** pp. 33–34)

54. B. Half-life = $0.693\ V_d/CL$, where V_d is the volume of distribution and CL is the clearance. Therefore,

$$T_{1/2} = \frac{0.693 \times 0.15 \text{ L/kg} \times 70 \text{ kg}}{48 \text{mL/min} \times 0.001 \text{ L/mL} \times 60 \text{ min/hr}} = 2.5 \text{ hr}$$

(**Ref. 1,** p. 40; **Ref. 4,** pp. 20–21; **Ref. 12,** p. 38)

55. E. Infusion rate = plasma concentration multiplied by clearance. Therefore, 15 µg/mL (48mL/min) = 720 µg/min. (**Ref. 1**, p. 43; **Ref. 4**, p. 29; **Ref. 12**, p. 42)

56. A. Loading dose = C_pV_d/F, where C_p is the desired plasma concentration, V_d is the volume of distribution, and F is the bioavailability. Therefore, loading dose = (10 µg/L)(100L/0.75). (**Ref. 1**, pp. 44–45; **Ref. 4**, p. 30; **Ref. 12**, pp. 43–44)

57. D. Biotransformation reactions usually yield compounds that are less lipophilic and more water soluble than the parent compounds. The more polar compounds diffuse less readily across tubular membranes, and consequently they are more readily excreted in the urine. Products may be pharmacologically more active or less active than parent compounds. (**Ref. 1**, p. 49; **Ref. 4**, pp. 13–14; **Ref. 12**, pp. 48–49)

58. C. Phase 2 reactions couple drugs or drug metabolites to endogenous substances such as glucuronic acid, sulfuric acid, acetic acid, or glycine to yield highly polar molecules. (**Ref. 1**, p. 54; **Ref. 4**, pp. 13–16; **Ref. 12**, pp. 53–54)

59. D. In humans, morphine is eliminated mainly by conjugation. (**Ref. 1**, pp. 54–55, 424; **Ref. 4**, pp. 14–15, 497; **Ref. 12**, p. 54)

60. A. Oxidation of phenobarbital into hydroxyphenobarbital accounts for most of the cessation of its action, though as much as 25% may be excreted by the kidneys. (**Ref. 1**, pp. 51–54, 309–310; **Ref. 4**, pp. 14–15; **Ref. 12**, pp. 50–52)

61. E. Approximately two thirds of digoxin is excreted unchanged by the kidneys. This accounts for its shorter duration of action as compared with digitoxin, which is metabolized mainly by the liver. (**Ref. 1**, pp. 178–179; **Ref. 4**, pp. 827–828; **Ref. 12**, p. 192)

62. A. Theophylline is oxidized in humans mainly by xanthine oxidase, but also by oxidative demethylation. (**Ref. 4**, p. 627)

63. C. The local anesthetic procaine is metabolized mainly by plasma and liver cholinesterases to water soluble metabolites that are excreted in the urine. (**Ref. 1**, p. 365; **Ref. 2**, p. 367; **Ref. 4**, p. 318; **Ref. 12**, p. 397)

64. D. Acetaminophen normally undergoes conjugation to glucuronide and sulfate derivatives, which comprise 95% of the total excreted products. (**Ref. 1,** p. 54–55; **Ref. 4,** p. 657; **Ref. 12,** p. 54)

65. A. Ethanol is oxidized to acetaldehyde in the liver mainly by alcohol dehydrogenase, but also by the mixed-function oxidase system. Acetaldehyde can be further oxidized in the liver to CO_2 and water. (**Ref. 1,** pp. 320–321; **Ref. 4,** p. 375; **Ref. 12,** pp. 350–351)

66. B. The tolbutamide package insert contains a warning about cardiotoxicity. The University Group Diabetes Program report suggested that tolbutamide has a toxic effect on the heart since some of the patients had heart attacks during their study. This might occur when a patient is given a large dose of tolbutamide. In patients with a genetic defect of ester hydrolysis, the tolbutamide would persist longer and a cumulative effect could occur, resulting in hypoglycemia and possibly cardiotoxicity. (**Ref. 1,** p. 596; **Ref. 4,** p. 1486; **Ref. 12,** p. 649)

67. C. Warfarin is an anticoagulant and a genetic defect in its inactivation would require the use of smaller than average doses of the drug. (**Ref. 1,** p. 56; **Ref. 4,** p. 73; **Ref. 12,** pp. 55–56)

68. A. Increased blood levels of isoniazid would lead to a variety of toxic effects on the nervous system including insomnia, muscle twitching, and peripheral neuritis. (**Ref. 1,** p. 654; **Ref. 4,** p. 1148; **Ref. 12,** pp. 708–709)

69. E. Succinylcholine was one of the first drugs discovered for which a genetic defect in metabolism greatly altered the drug's use. A defect in pseudocholinesterase resulted in prolonging the action of succinylcholine from minutes to hours. (**Ref. 1,** p. 56; **Ref. 8,** p. 73; **Ref. 12,** pp. 55–56)

70. D. Debrisoquin is an antihypertensive-vasodilator drug. When the blood levels of the drug are increased due to a genetic defect in oxidation, the side effect is orthostatic hypotension. (**Ref. 1,** p. 56; **Ref. 12,** pp. 55–56)

2

Water, Electrolytes, and Diuretics

DIRECTIONS (Questions 71–78): Each of the questions or incomplete statements below is followed by five suggested answers or completions. Select the **one** that is best in each case.

---

71. All of the following statements about furosemide are correct EXCEPT
    A. toxic effects are unusual, but include gastrointestinal distress, skin rash, thrombocytopenia, neutropenia, and hypochloremia
    B. its primary effect is inhibition of chloride reabsorption in the ascending limb of the loop of Henle
    C. it may produce hypovolemic shock due to an exaggerated response
    D. it is one of the most potent diuretic drugs
    E. when given in high doses it may produce metabolic acidosis because it inhibits H^+ secretion in the distal tubule

72. Undesirable side effects of thiazide diuretics include all of the following EXCEPT
    A. with prolonged use, azotemia may occur
    B. hyperglycemia
    C. reduced renal blood flow and glomerular filtration rate
    D. potassium retention with excess water loss
    E. cholestatic hepatitis

73. All of the following statements about mannitol are correct EXCEPT
   A. it produces diuresis in the presence of reduced glomerular filtration rate
   B. it is filterable and poorly reabsorbed in the renal tubules
   C. it produces very little, if any, change in the acid-base balance
   D. it is used to measure the rate of glomerular filtration
   E. it is the diuretic of choice to treat chronic pulmonary edema

74. Which of the following diuretics is most apt to cause hyperkalemia?
   A. Chlorothiazide
   B. Triamterene
   C. Furosemide
   D. Acetazolamide
   E. Mannitol

75. Carbonic anhydrase inhibitors
   A. cause an increase in intraocular pressure
   B. induce epileptic seizures
   C. have prolonged duration of action
   D. cause irreversible inhibition of carbonic anhydrase
   E. produce a marked increase in potassium ion secretion

76. Contraindications for the use of thiazides include all of the following EXCEPT
   A. hepatic encephalopathy
   B. renal insufficiency
   C. hepatic cirrhosis
   D. nephrogenic diabetes insipidus
   E. digitalis-induced hypokalemia

77. Antidiuretic hormone (ADH)
   A. is orally effective
   B. is used for treatment of diabetes insipidus
   C. is usually only given for a short period of time
   D. causes vasoconstriction in doses that produce antidiuresis
   E. usually causes coronary vasodilation

78. Which of the following statements is INCORRECT?
   A. Restriction of sodium chloride intake inhibits the antidiuretic effect of thiazides in diabetes insipidus

   B. Thiazides are effective in treating diabetes insipidus
   C. Patients may have allergic reactions to vasopressin
   D. Vasopressin and ADH are the same compound
   E. Thiazides may reduce the urine volume to 50% of pretreatment values in diabetes insipidus

---

DIRECTIONS (Questions 79–91): The group of questions below consists of five lettered headings followed by a list of numbered words or phrases. For each numbered word or phrase, select the **one** lettered heading that is most closely associated with it. Each lettered heading may be selected once, more than once, or not at all.

Questions 79–83:
   A. Mannitol
   B. Ethacrynic acid
   C. Acetazolamide
   D. Chlorothiazide
   E. Spironolactone

79. Greatest increase in urinary sodium chloride

80. Decreased urinary bicarbonate elimination with a large increase in urinary excretion of sodium

81. Produces a large increase in urinary bicarbonate

82. Minimal effect on urinary potassium

83. Used in combination with loop diuretics to decrease toxicity

Questions 84–87:
   A. hydrochlorothiazide
   B. nifedipine
   C. verapamil
   D. probenecid
   E. mannitol

84. Major use is for edema associated with head injury

85. A calcium-channel blocker used for its vasodilatory effect

86. A diuretic used for hypercalciuria

87. Inhibitor of organic acid transport

Questions 88–91:
   A. Glomerulus
   B. Proximal tubule
   C. Loop of Henle
   D. Distal tubule
   E. Collecting tubule

88. Triamterene

89. Vasopressin on the V_2 receptors of the kidney

90. Carbonic anhydrase inhibitors (bicarbonate action)

91. Hydrochlorothiazide

Water, Electrolytes, and Diuretics

Answers and Discussion

71. E. Furosemide and ethacrynic acid, known as high-ceiling or loop diuretics, can produce metabolic alkalosis, not acidosis; they are excreted mainly in the urine by the proximal tubules and inhibit sodium and chloride reabsorption in the ascending loop of Henle. **(Ref. 1,** p. 219; **Ref. 2,** pp. 226–228; **Ref. 4,** pp. 721–724; **Ref. 12,** pp. 238–239)

72. D. Hypokalemia, not hyperkalemia, is the most common adverse effect of the thiazides. To keep the potassium levels normal, therapy should include one or more of the following: (1) diet rich in fruits and vegetables, (2) potassium chloride taken orally daily, or (3) combination with potassium-sparing diuretics. **(Ref. 1,** p. 221; **Ref. 2,** p. 224; **Ref. 4,** p. 721; **Ref. 12,** p. 240)

73. E. Because mannitol must be given intravenously, its use as a diuretic is very limited. Administered as a hypertonic solution, it reduces elevated intracranial pressure without a rebound increase in pressure; it also increases the extracellular volume so its use is contraindicated in patients with cardiac decompensation. **(Ref. 1,** pp. 224–225; **Ref. 2,** pp. 221–222; **Ref. 4,** pp. 714–715; **Ref. 12,** p. 243)

74. B. Triamterene and spironolactone are considered potassium-sparing agents. Triamterene promotes sodium excretion and spironolactone is an aldosterone antagonist. They may cause hyperkalemia. **(Ref. 1,** pp. 222–223; **Ref. 2,** pp. 224–225; **Ref. 4,** pp. 725–727; **Ref. 12,** p. 241)

75. E. The effects or actions of carbonic anhydrase inhibitors are the opposite of choices A through D. Intraocular pressure is reduced, epilepsy can be managed on a short-term basis, the compounds have a limited duration of action, and they are reversible inhibitors. **(Ref. 1,** pp. 215–216; **Ref. 2,** p. 222; **Ref. 4,** pp. 716–717; **Ref. 12,** pp. 236–237)

76. D. Thiazides may produce antidiuresis in patients who are not responsive to ADH. The action is potentiated by dietary sodium restriction. **(Ref. 1,** p. 221; **Ref. 2,** p. 224; **Ref. 4,** p. 721; **Ref. 12,** p. 239)

77. B. Vasopressin for the treatment of diabetes insipidus requires life-long therapy. It is a peptide and thus rapidly inactivated by trypsin. Large doses are required for vasoconstriction but the compound is contraindicated in patients with coronary artery disease. **(Ref. 1,** p. 257; **Ref. 2,** p. 729; **Ref. 4,** pp. 739–740; **Ref. 12,** pp. 574–575)

78. A. Paradoxically, thiazides and ethacrynic acid may be used in patients with diabetes insipidus who are resistant to ADH. Sodium chloride restriction may enhance the effectiveness. **(Ref. 2,** p. 221; **Ref. 4,** p. 741; **Ref. 12,** p. 247)

79. B. Ethacrynic acid and furosemide have actions in the thick ascending loop of Henle to inhibit sodium chloride reabsorption. An intense diuresis with a high level of sodium excretion is characteristic of these agents. **(Ref. 1,** pp. 217, 225; **Ref. 12,** p. 238)

80. B. Due to the increased salt and water delivered to the distal segments of the nephron, enhanced potassium and hydrogen ion secretion results. This leads to metabolic alkalosis. **(Ref. 1,** p. 219; **Ref. 12,** pp. 238–239)

81. C. Carbonic anhydrase inhibitors are effective for a short period but cause a large elimination of bicarbonate ion. They depress bicarbonate reabsorption in the proximal tubule. **(Ref. 1,** pp. 216, 225; **Ref. 12,** p. 235)

82. E. Spironolactone is a potassium-sparing diuretic that inhibits mineralocorticoids by combining with mineralocorticoid receptors. These agents act in the collecting tubules and ducts. (**Ref. 1,** pp. 223, 225; **Ref. 12,** p. 241)

83. D. The use of a thiazide with a loop diuretic decreases the potential for ototoxicity. This combination is also effective in refractory edema and reduces the reliance on large doses of loop agents. (**Ref. 1,** pp. 221–222; **Ref. 12,** p. 244)

84. E. Mannitol is an osmotic diuretic that reduces body water, not ions. This action is useful when head-injury–induced cerebral edema occurs in cases where intraocular pressure is increased. (**Ref. 1,** p. 224; **Ref. 2,** pp. 221–222; **Ref. 4,** pp. 714–715; **Ref. 12,** p. 243)

85. B. Nifedipine and verapamil are both calcium channel blockers capable of causing vasodilation. Nifedipine is used for its vasodilating action in treating hypertension. Verapamil is used to inhibit AV conduction in the myocardium to protect the ventricle from aberrant electrical activity occurring in the atrium. (**Ref. 1,** p. 155; **Ref. 2,** pp. 251–252; **Ref. 4,** p. 777; **Ref. 12,** p. 163)

86. A. The two diuretics listed are mannitol and hydrochlorothiazide. Mannitol is an osmotic diuretic. The thiazides are useful in managing increased calcium levels and preventing formation of stones. (**Ref. 1,** p. 221; **Ref. 4,** p. 721; **Ref. 12,** pp. 667–668)

87. D. Probenecid reduces the elimination of organic acids in the urine. Penicillin and related antibiotics have decreased elimination. Uric acid, on the other hand, needs to be reabsorbed, so probenecid causes a uricosuric effect. (**Ref. 1,** p. 508; **Ref. 2,** pp. 505, 559; **Ref. 4,** p. 745; **Ref. 12,** p. 554)

88. D. Triamterene, by its action on the distal tubules, inhibits sodium reabsorption and potassium secretion. Therefore, in combination with the thiazides, triamterene prevents the hypokalemic effects of the thiazides. (**Ref. 1,** p. 223; **Ref. 2,** 226; **Ref. 4,** p. 727; **Ref. 12,** p. 241)

89. E. Vasopressin acting on the V_2 receptors in the collecting tubules causes them to become permeable to water. Because the urine at this site is hypotonic, water is reabsorbed by osmosis. (**Ref. 1,** p. 526; **Ref. 2,** pp. 214–215; **Ref. 4,** pp. 736, 737; **Ref. 12,** pp. 574–575)

90. **B.** The major action of carbonic anhydrase inhibitors is to inhibit bicarbonate reabsorption in the proximal tubule brush border. These agents also alter H^+ secretion in the distal tubule and collecting duct. (**Ref. 1,** p. 215; **Ref. 2,** p. 222; **Ref. 4,** p. 716; **Ref. 12,** p. 235)

91. **D.** The major site of action of hydrochlorothiazide is the distal portion of the ascending limb of the distal tubule. (**Ref. 1,** p. 220; **Ref. 2,** p. 223; **Ref. 4,** pp. 718–719; **Ref. 12,** p. 239)

3

Drugs Affecting the Autonomic Nervous System

DIRECTIONS (Questions 92–127): Each of the questions or incomplete statements below is followed by five suggested answers or completions. Select the **one** that is best in each case.

---

92. The mechanism of action of prazosin involves
    A. activation of β_1-receptors
    B. specific activation of α_2-receptors
    C. blockade of α_1-receptors
    D. elimination of β_2 effects
    E. nonequilibrium α-adrenergic blockade

93. The distinguishing feature of nadolol among the β-adrenergic blocking agents is
    A. cardioselectivity
    B. β_2 selectivity
    C. duration of action ($t^{\frac{1}{2}}$)
    D. nonequilibrium blockade
    E. intrinsic sympathomimetic activity

94. Noncatecholamine adrenergic amines differ from catecholamines in that they
- **A.** have a short duration of action
- **B.** are not effective if administered orally
- **C.** do not act indirectly, but usually combine directly with adrenergic receptors of the α_1 and β_2 subtypes
- **D.** tend to have greater central nervous system (CNS) effects following oral administration
- **E.** are metabolized at a more rapid rate

95. Adrenergic amines might be employed therapeutically for all of the following conditions EXCEPT
- **A.** relief of symptoms of acute hypersensitivity reactions to drugs
- **B.** production of miosis and cycloplegia
- **C.** narcolepsy
- **D.** activation of the vagal reflex mechanism in paroxysmal atrial tachycardia
- **E.** reduction of nasal congestion for temporary relief from upper respiratory infections

$$- \qquad +$$

Acetylcholinesterase

anionic site   esteratic site

96. Above is a diagrammatic representation of sites of drug interaction on the acetylcholinesterase enzyme. All of the following statements are true EXCEPT
- **A.** acetylcholine is hydrolyzed after combination with the esteratic (+) and anionic (−) sites
- **B.** neostigmine carbamylates the esteratic (+) site and is slowly hydrolyzed
- **C.** irreversible inhibitors of the enzyme act by forming an alkyl-phosphorylation of the anionic site (−)
- **D.** regeneration of the enzyme occurs when oximes attach to the anionic site (−) and exert a nucleophilic attack on the phosphorus
- **E.** the binding of diisopropyl fluorophosphate (DFP) to the esteratic site (+) undergoes an "aging" process

97. Postoperative urinary retention may be best treated with
   A. DFP
   B. carbachol
   C. ephedrine
   D. bethanechol
   E. atropine

98. The enhanced pressor response to norepinephrine in humans after the administration of amitriptyline is most likely caused by
   A. increased sensitivity of tissue to norepinephrine
   B. increased activity of catechol-O-methyltransferase (COMT)
   C. interference with uptake of norepinephrine into adrenergic nerves
   D. increased activity of monoamine oxidase
   E. decreased destruction of norepinephrine by metabolic enzymes

99. The major pathway of the removal of norepinephrine released from nerves into the synaptic gap is
   A. degradation by monoamine oxidase
   B. uptake into adrenergic nerves (uptake$_1$)
   C. diffusion from the synapse into the general circulation
   D. binding with plasma proteins
   E. uptake into smooth muscle cells of spleen, heart, and kidney (uptake$_2$)

100. Which of the following is an accepted therapeutic use of epinephrine?
   A. Combinations with local anesthetics in 1:1000 concentrations
   B. Treatment of pheochromocytoma
   C. IV infusion in cases of hemorrhagic shock
   D. Treatment of cardiac asthma
   E. Treatment of acute hypersensitivity reaction to drugs

101. Timolol
   A. is an anticholinesterase
   B. is a cholinergic drug
   C. is a β-adrenergic antagonist
   D. is principally an α-adrenergic agonist with minimal β-adrenergic agonist activity
   E. causes mydriasis and ciliary spasm fixed for near vision

102. The mechanism of action of hemicholinium is due to
    A. prevention of the liberation of acetylcholine (ACH)
    B. mimicry of the action of ACH
    C. blocking of the transport system responsible for choline accumulation in terminals of cholinergic fibers
    D. inactivation of cholinesterase
    E. prevention of the interaction between ACH and the receptor sites

103. The mechanism of action of botulinum toxin is
    A. mimicry of ACH
    B. prevention of release of ACH
    C. potentiation of action of cholinesterase
    D. inhibition of action of cholinesterase
    E. prevention of the synthesis of ACH

104. Which of the following statements is true regarding sympathomimetic amines?
    A. Phenylephrine or methoxamine may successfully end attacks of paroxysmal atrial or nodal tachycardia by vagal reflex without causing significant cardiac stimulation
    B. The pressor action of metaraminol is mainly indirect and is dependent upon epinephrine release
    C. Isoproterenol and dobutamine are typical α-receptor stimulators
    D. The injection of epinephrine will cause a marked decrease in plasma free fatty acids, but only in the presence of a functioning adrenal gland
    E. Epinephrine produces an increase in coronary blood flow, which accounts for its usefulness in relieving precordial pain in anginal attacks

105. Regarding the treatment of Parkinson's disease, all of the following statements are true EXCEPT
    A. the parkinsonian patient has a reduced amount of dopamine in basal ganglia
    B. reserpine depletes dopamine and may produce parkinsonian symptoms
    C. phenothiazines antagonize catecholamines and cause parkinsonian side effects
    D. dopamine readily crosses the blood-brain barrier
    E. impressive improvement occurs in patients with L-dopa in the first few years of treatment but is often not sustained

106. All of the following statements are true concerning the "amine pump," or uptake mechanism, of the adrenergic nerve terminals EXCEPT
  A. it is not highly specific for norepinephrine
  B. it will take up metaraminol in significant amounts
  C. it will take up and accumulate "false transmitters"
  D. it will not take up 6-hydroxydopamine
  E. it is blocked by imipramine

107. Which of the following statements concerning nicotinic and muscarinic receptors is FALSE?
  A. Nicotine has the property of being both a cholinergic receptor stimulant and a blocking agent
  B. The nicotinic receptors of autonomic ganglia and skeletal muscle are not entirely identical
  C. It is now accepted that autonomic ganglion cells have both nicotinic and muscarinic receptors
  D. Atropine blocks the excitatory muscarinic actions of acetylcholine, but not the inhibitory actions
  E. Pirenzepine selectively inhibits M_1 muscarinic receptors in the ganglion

108. All of the following are α-adrenergic blockers EXCEPT
  A. ergotamine
  B. prazosin
  C. ergonovine
  D. phenoxybenzamine
  E. phentolamine

109. All of the following are typical cholinergic effects EXCEPT
  A. a decrease in heart rate
  B. an increase in atrioventricular (AV) conduction time
  C. an increase in secretion of sweat
  D. an increase in pupillary diameter
  E. a contraction of bronchial muscle

110. Acetylcholine is the neurotransmitter at all of the following sites EXCEPT
   A. muscarinic receptor sites
   B. nicotinic$_1$ receptor sites
   C. nicotinic$_2$ receptor sites
   D. adrenergic ganglia
   E. α_2-adrenergic receptor sites

111. The process referred to as uptake$_2$
   A. is inhibited by cocaine
   B. causes decreased release of norepinephrine
   C. is also called extraneuronal uptake
   D. is blocked by imipramine
   E. blocks the action of tyramine

112. All of the following statements are true regarding nicotine EXCEPT
   A. nicotine is an alkaloid that is readily absorbed through the skin
   B. nicotine both stimulates and blocks receptor sites
   C. the action of nicotine is limited to skeletal muscle paralysis
   D. the effects of toxic doses of nicotine can be predicted by knowing the predominant innervation of an organ
   E. administration of nicotine would be expected to cause release of epinephrine from the adrenal gland

113. Administration of an infusion of norepinephrine to a person will result in
   A. an increase in peripheral resistance
   B. a decrease in AV transmission
   C. an increase in heart rate
   D. a decrease in mean blood pressure
   E. a decrease in diastolic blood pressure

114. Epinephrine
   A. is a potent stimulant of respiration
   B. inhibits the release of inflammatory mediators from mast cells
   C. causes airway smooth muscle to contract
   D. may cause hypoglycemia
   E. produces miosis

115. Desensitization to catecholamines may be caused by all of the following EXCEPT
   A. phosphorylation of receptors
   B. internalization of receptors
   C. alteration of G proteins
   D. alterations in cyclic nucleotide phosphodiesterase
   E. stimulation or acceleration of cAMP production

116. Human uterine smooth muscle
   A. is relaxed by muscarinic receptor activation
   B. is relaxed by α-adrenergic receptor activation
   C. may be relaxed by β_2-receptor activation at parturition
   D. can be inhibited by α-receptor activation
   E. relaxes when β_2 agonists are given to nonpregnant patients

117. Dopamine
   A. causes renal vasodilation through D_1-receptors
   B. reduces peripheral resistance when administered in high concentrations
   C. has minimal β_1 effects on the heart
   D. inactivates adenylyl cyclase
   E. rapidly enters the CNS

118. β_2-adrenergic agonists
   A. cause significant skeletal muscle relaxation as a side effect
   B. produce reduced levels of glucose in the blood
   C. cause arrhythmias in most patients
   D. may cause the insulin requirement to increase in diabetic patients
   E. cause significant and troublesome tolerance in most patients

119. Ipratropium
   A. is a bronchoconstrictor
   B. must be administered orally
   C. should not be given to asthmatic patients
   D. is a quaternary compound
   E. usually causes excessive salivation

120. In the following list all are correct pairings EXCEPT
   A. labetalol/lack of α_2 activity
   B. pindolol/intrinsic sympathomimetic activity
   C. bitolterol/prodrug
   D. tyramine/indirectly-acting amine
   E. metoprolol/selective β_2 agonist

121. Antimuscarinic agents
   A. are difficult to use without troublesome side effects
   B. effectively decrease gastric acid secretion in low doses
   C. produce mydriasis without cycloplegia
   D. can be given to produce cycloplegia without mydriasis
   E. are relatively nontoxic and can be safely employed in large doses

122. Cholinergic excess
   A. may occur as a result of ingestion of the mushroom, *Amanita phalloides*
   B. in the central nervous system (CNS) can be effectively treated with ipratropium
   C. caused by organophosphates can be reversed if pralidoxime is administered immediately after organophosphate ingestion
   D. is almost always produced by ingestion of *Amanita muscaria*
   E. in the CNS is treated with pralidoxime

123. Regarding anticholinesterase activity, all of the following statements are true EXCEPT
   A. neostigmine is a quaternary amine
   B. physostigmine enters into the CNS
   C. both neostigmine and physostigmine inhibit the hydrolysis of acetylcholine
   D. neostigmine can cause direct cholinergic activation of skeletal muscle nicotinic receptors
   E. neostigmine and physostigmine are considered to be irreversible agents

124. Regarding cholinoceptive sites
   A. actions of acetylcholine are potentiated by scopolamine
   B. bethanechol is potentiated by neostigmine
   C. curare will inhibit the effectiveness of neostigmine at the neuromuscular junction

    D. hexamethonium is a neuromuscular blocker
    E. muscarinic receptors are not considered cholinoceptive

125. All of the following statements are true for pilocarpine EXCEPT
    A. causes contraction of the intestinal tract
    B. may be used to treat asthma
    C. induces vasodilation
    D. is effective for open-angle glaucoma
    E. produces marked diaphoresis (sweating)

126. The effects of acetylcholine or cholinergic agonists on the myocardium include
    A. counteraction of the indirect effect of digitalis
    B. decreased contractile force development
    C. decreased AV conduction time
    D. stimulation of the sinoatrial (SA) node
    E. increased speed of AV conduction

127. Ganglionic blockade would most likely produce
    A. increased urinary frequency
    B. decreased heart rate
    C. salivation
    D. mydriasis
    E. vasoconstriction

Questions 128 and 129: In Figure 2, the blood pressure graphic record obtained from a dog anesthetized with pentobarbital shows the effect of 10 µg/kg of acetylcholine given intravenously at A and at B followed by 100 µg/kg of acetylcholine given intravenously at C and at D.
    A. Atropine
    B. Ephedrine
    C. Epinephrine
    D. Phentolamine
    E. Phenylephrine

128. From the preceding list of drugs, select the one given between injections A and B (Figure 2)

129. From the preceding list of drugs, select the one given between injections C and D (Figure 2)

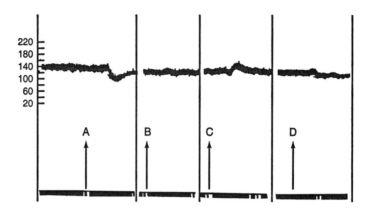

Figure 2 Blood pressure record from dog anesthetized with sodium pentobarbital showing the effects of intravenous injections of acetylcholine 10 µg/kg at A and B and 100 µg/kg at C and D. (Adapted from Goth A: *Medical Pharmacology*, 11th Ed. St. Louis, CV Mosby, 1984, with permission.)

Questions 130 and 131: The blood pressure graphic record shown in Figure 3 was obtained from a dog anesthetized with pentobarbital.

    A. Atropine
    B. Ephedrine
    C. Epinephrine
    D. Phentolamine
    E. Phenylephrine

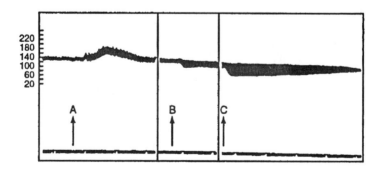

Figure 3 (Adapted from Goth A: *Medical Pharmacology*, 11th Ed. St. Louis, CV Mosby, 1984, with permission.)

130. From the preceding list of drugs, select the one given at A in Figure 3 where time intervals are shown in minutes

131. The drug given at A was injected again at C in the same dosage; from the preceding list of drugs, select the one given at B (Figure 3)

DIRECTIONS (Questions 132–134): Each group of questions below consists of five lettered headings followed by a list of numbered words, phrases, or statements. For each numbered word, phrase, or statement, select the **one** lettered heading that is most closely associated with it. Each lettered heading may be selected once, more than once, or not at all.

Questions 132–134:
- **A.** Phentolamine
- **B.** Prazosin
- **C.** Phenoxybenzamine
- **D.** Clonidine
- **E.** Yohimbine

132. An adrenergic-blocking agent that has a long duration of action and is relatively α_1-receptor selective.

133. A selective antagonist of α_2-adrenergic receptors

134. An α_1-adrenergic receptor antagonist used for hypertension

Questions 135–139:
- **A.** Propranolol
- **B.** Haloperidol
- **C.** Chlorpromazine
- **D.** Ergonovine
- **E.** Pindolol

135. A nonselective β-adrenergic–blocking agent with intrinsic sympathomimetic activity

136. This compound possesses significant membrane-stabilizing effects

137. This neuroleptic compound blocks dopamine receptors specifically

138. This alkaloid causes contraction of uterine smooth muscle

139. This agent has been shown to prevent recurrence of myocardial infarction and to decrease mortality

Questions 140–143:
- **A.** Ganglionic blocking agent
- **B.** β-adrenergic–blocking agent
- **C.** α-adrenergic–blocking agent
- **D.** Neuronal blocking agent
- **E.** Muscarinic blocking agent

140. Trimetaphan

141. Metyrosine

142. Metoprolol

143. Bretylium

Questions 144–146:
- **A.** Neostigmine
- **B.** Cocaine
- **C.** Tranylcypromine
- **D.** Propranolol
- **E.** Pindolol

144. Administration of this local anesthetic compound would potentiate the action of exogenously administered epinephrine

145. A side effect might be excessive salivation

146. Use of this agent must be discontinued slowly

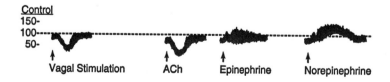

147. If the response below is obtained, the drug administered after the control sequence above was

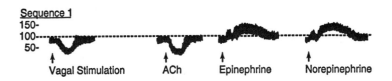

Sequence 1

A. a ganglionic blocker
B. a β-adrenergic antagonist
C. a cholinesterase inhibitor
D. an α-adrenergic antagonist
E. a cholinergic antagonist

148. If the response below is obtained, the drug administered after the previous control sequence was:

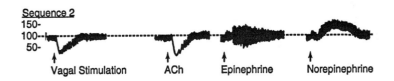

Sequence 2

A. a ganglionic blocker
B. a β-adrenergic antagonist
C. a cholinesterase inhibitor
D. an α-adrenergic antagonist
E. a cholinergic antagonist

DIRECTIONS (Questions 149–151): Each of the questions or incomplete statements below is followed by five suggested answers or completions. Select the **one** that is best in each case.

---

149. The correct profile for receptor activation by epinephrine is
A. $\alpha_1, \alpha_2, \beta_1, \beta_2$
B. $\alpha_1, \alpha_2, \beta_1$
C. α_1, α_2
D. $\alpha_1, \beta_1, \beta_2$
E. β_1, β_2

150. In selecting an agent to elicit an increase in peripheral resistance without direct cardiac effects, the agent of choice would be
A. norepinephrine
B. dopamine
C. phenylephrine
D. phentolamine
E. propranolol

151. Indirectly acting adrenergic amines
A. release norepinephrine from extraneuronal sites.
B. release catecholamines from storage granules
C. inhibit the action of directly acting adrenergic amines
D. release catecholamines from cytoplasmic storage sites
E. are potentiated by tricyclic antidepressants

DIRECTIONS (Questions 152–164): Each group of questions below consists of five lettered headings followed by a list of numbered words, phrases, or statements. For each numbered word, phrase, or statement, select the **one** lettered heading that is most closely associated with it. Each lettered heading may be selected once, more than once, or not at all.

Questions 152–154:
A. Acetylcholine
B. Carbachol
C. Bethanechol
D. Methacholine
E. Choline

152. Agent predominately used for its cardiovascular effects

153. Resistant to inhibition by atropine and not hydrolyzed by cholinesterases

154. Not employed therapeutically because of its rapid hydrolysis and lack of specificity

Questions 155–157:
A. Muscarinic agonists
B. Anticholinergic agents
C. Ganglionic blocking drugs

    D. Nicotinic agonists
    E. Nicotinic antagonists

155. Contraindications include asthma, coronary insufficiency, and peptic ulcer

156. Signs of toxicity may include hot, dry skin and delirium

157. Stimulates both skeletal muscle and ganglionic sites

Questions 158–160:
    A. Cromolyn
    B. Minoxidil
    C. Timolol
    D. Methyldopa
    E. Propranolol

158. Useful in the prevention of migraine headaches

159. Useful to prevent attacks of asthma, but ineffective if the asthmatic episode is occurring

160. Side actions and toxic effects include fluid retention, excessive hair growth on the face and back, and pericardial effusion

Questions 161–163:
    A. Pilocarpine
    B. Mecamylamine
    C. Timolol
    D. Metoprolol
    E. Clonidine

161. A nonselective β-adrenergic antagonist useful in the treatment of glaucoma

162. Useful in treatment of glaucoma; drug causes miosis and spasm of the ciliary muscles

163. Useful in treating hypertension because of its CNS effects

DIRECTIONS (Questions 164–168): Each of the questions or incomplete statements below is followed by five suggested answers or completions. Select the **one** that is best in each case.

164. The use of amphetamine-type compounds for obesity
    A. is highly effective
    B. is based on suppression of the lateral hypothalamic feeding center
    C. causes stimulation of the ventromedial satiety center
    D. produces major increases in metabolic rate
    E. is beneficial once an initial increase in weight occurs

165. Blockade of this receptor would lead to increased levels of catecholamines in the neuroeffector junction.
    A. α_1
    B. α_2
    C. β_1
    D. β_2
    E. Dopamine

166. All of the following statements about propranolol are true EXCEPT
    A. propranolol must be withdrawn slowly
    B. propranolol undergoes first-pass metabolism
    C. propranolol exerts a primary antiarrhythmic action due to membrane stabilization
    D. propranolol does not block α-receptors
    E. propranolol is not a selective β-adrenergic blocker

167. Direct actions of acetylcholine include all of the following EXCEPT
    A. miosis
    B. vasodilation
    C. bradycardia
    D. inhibition of EDRF
    E. contraction of urinary bladder sphincter

168. All of the following statements about cholinesterase inhibitors are correct EXCEPT
   A. edrophonium is a reversible inhibitor with a brief duration of action
   B. organophosphate inhibitors covalently bind to the enzyme
   C. neostigmine phosphorylates the enzyme
   D. pralidoximes are reactivators of the enzyme
   E. reactivation is possible if the enzyme inhibitor complex has not "aged"

Drugs Affecting the Autonomic Nervous System

Answers and Discussion

92. C. Prazosin is a unique antihypertensive agent which reduces blood pressure by selectively blocking α_1 receptors. (**Ref. 1,** p. 127; **Ref. 2,** p. 136; **Ref. 3,** p. 161; **Ref. 4,** p. 226; **Ref. 12,** p. 135)

93. C. Nadolol has a half-life of 14 to 18 hours, is a nonselective β-adrenergic blocker, and does not activate β receptors. (**Ref. 1,** p. 132; **Ref. 4,** p. 234; **Ref. 12,** p. 139)

94. D. Noncatecholamines are resistant to enzymatic inactivation by monoamine oxidase (MAO) or catechol-O-methyltransferase (COMT), leading to a longer duration of action, oral effectiveness, and penetration into the CNS, causing stimulation. Much of the action of these compounds is a result of releasing norepinephrine from adrenergic nerve endings. See discussion of amphetamine or ephedrine. (**Ref. 1,** p. 118; **Ref. 2,** p. 117; **Ref. 4,** pp. 188–190; **Ref. 12,** p. 125)

95. B. Adrenergic amines can be employed to produce mydriasis without cycloplegia. Paralysis of accommodation, or cycloplegia, is caused by anticholinergic agents, such as atropine. (**Ref. 1,** pp. 120–121; **Ref. 2,** p. 125; **Ref. 3,** p. 146; **Ref. 4,** p. 217; **Ref. 6,** p. 177; **Ref. 12,** pp. 127–128)

96. C. Both the carbamyl ester and the organophosphate-type anti-cholinesterase agents covalently bind to the enzyme. Phosphorylation occurs at the esteratic site. Enzyme function is restored over time, with carbamate hydrolysis occurring more rapidly. (**Ref. 1**, pp. 90–91; **Ref. 2**, p. 163; **Ref. 4**, pp. 132–134· **Ref. 12**, pp. 95–97)

97. D. Bethanechol is useful in treating postoperative, postpartum, and neurogenic urinary retention through its muscarinic agonistic actions on smooth muscle of the urinary bladder. Carbachol is less specific. (**Ref. 1**, p. 92; **Ref. 3**, p. 104; **Ref. 4**, pp. 126–127; **Ref. 12**, p. 98)

98. C. Amitriptyline, through its cocaine-like action, blocks the transport system in the axonal membrane of the adrenergic nerve terminal, resulting in an accumulation of norepinephrine at extracellular sites. (**Ref. 1**, p. 79; **Ref. 2**, p. 114; **Ref. 4**, p. 413; **Ref. 12**, p. 74)

99. B. The principle mechanism for the termination of adrenergic action appears to be the reuptake of adrenergic neurotransmitter at postganglionic sympathetic nerve terminals. This energy-dependent process is termed uptake$_1$ to distinguish it from uptake$_2$, which is an extraneuronal process. Uptake is primarily a removal process, since synthesis of transmitter can adequately replenish the store. (**Ref. 1**, p. 74; **Ref. 2**, p. 110; **Ref. 4**, p. 106; **Ref. 12**, p. 76)

100. E. Epinephrine, 1:1000, is a time-honored drug used in the treatment of acute hypersensitivity reactions to drugs and other allergens. It is also widely used with local anesthetics to delay absorption and prolong anesthesia; however, concentrations of 1:200,000 to 1:100,000 are employed for this purpose. (**Ref. 1**, pp. 120–121; **Ref. 2**, pp. 120–124; **Ref. 3**, p. 147; **Ref. 4**, pp. 214–218; **Ref. 12**, pp. 127–128)

101. C. Timolol is a nonselective β-adrenergic antagonist useful in treatment of hypertension and glaucoma. Recently, timolol has been approved for treatment of certain cardiovascular diseases. Note that the USAN, U.S. adopted names, for β-adrenergic blockers end in -olol. (**Ref. 1**, p.132; **Ref. 3**, p. 166; **Ref. 4**, p. 235; **Ref. 6**, p. 550; **Ref. 12**, p. 141)

102. C. All are mechanisms that can influence cholinergic activity. (See tables in references.) Hemicholinium limits the available choline, thereby restricting or preventing the synthesis and storage of acetylcholine. (**Ref. 1**, p. 79; **Ref. 2**, p. 114; **Ref. 3**, p. 89; **Ref. 4**, pp. 96, 114; **Ref. 12**, p. 84)

103. B. Botulinum toxin prevents the release of acetylcholine not only in the ganglia but at all cholinergic sites. Death is generally due to respiratory failure. (**Ref. 1**, p. 79; **Ref. 2**, p. 114; **Ref. 3**, pp. 91, 98; **Ref. 4**, p. 97; **Ref. 12**, p. 84)

104. A. Upon intravenous administration of either phenylephrine or methoxamine (both potent vasoconstrictors with little cardiac stimulatory activity), the elicited pressor response initiates vagal reflexes often capable of terminating paroxysmal atrial tachycardia. Metaraminol is primarily direct acting. Epinephrine increases plasma free fatty acids and may cause anginal pain due to its positive inotropic and chronotropic effects on the heart. Isoproterenol and dobutamine are β agonists. (**Ref. 1**, p. 120; **Ref. 2**, p. 126; **Ref. 4**, pp. 208, 216; **Ref. 12**, p. 128)

105. D. Since dopamine does not cross the blood-brain barrier efficiently, its precursor, L-dopa, which readily enters the brain, is widely used in the treatment of parkinsonism. In current practice, levodopa is almost always administered with a peripheral inhibitor of dopa decarboxylase (carbidopa). (**Ref. 1**, pp. 383–385; **Ref. 3**, pp. 288–291; **Ref. 4**, pp. 466, 472; **Ref. 12**, pp. 420–421)

106. D. Injurious compounds such as 6-hydroxydopamine (6-OH-DA) are readily taken up by the nerve-membrane amine pump and lead to destruction of the sympathetic nerve endings. (**Ref. 1**, p. 79; **Ref. 3**, pp. 96, 97; **Ref. 12**, p. 84)

107. D. Atropine, a muscarinic cholinergic blocking agent, blocks all the muscarinic effects of acetylcholine, whether they are excitatory or inhibitory. Nicotine initially stimulates and then blocks. In the periphery it acts on two separate types of receptors, called nicotine ganglionic and nicotinic neuromuscular. (**Ref. 1**, p. 82; **Ref. 2**, pp. 153, 172; **Ref. 4**, pp. 153, 180, 181; **Ref. 12**, p. 88)

108. C. Although ergotamine possesses appreciable α-adrenergic blocking properties, this action is not shared by ergonovine because it lacks the polypeptide side chain necessary for the α-blocking activity in ergot alkaloids. Ergonovine is used for postpartum hemorrhage, while ergotamine is used to diagnose migraine headache. Prazosin is an α_1 selective blocker, phenoxybenzamine is a nonequilibrium α blocker, and phentolamine is a nonselective α blocker. **(Ref. 3, pp. 162, 597; Ref. 4, pp. 942, 943)**

109. D. The typical effect of cholinergic agents on the pupil is one of miosis. This effect is caused by a contraction of the circular smooth muscle of the iris, which is under parasympathetic control. **(Ref. 1, p. 77; Ref. 2, p. 147; Ref. 4, pp. 89, 127; Ref. 12, p. 81)**

110. E. Acetylcholine is the mediator in all ganglia, at skeletal muscle neuromuscular junctions, and at all postganglionic parasympathetic fibers. Adrenergic receptors have norepinephrine as the mediator. **(Ref. 1, pp. 71–72; Ref. 2, p. 112; Ref. 3, p. 85; Ref. 4, pp. 97–98; Ref. 12, p. 74)**

111. C. Uptake$_2$ is an extraneuronal process that may be more important for circulating catecholamines. It is inhibited by glucocorticoids. Cocaine and imipramine inhibit uptake$_1$ while norepinephrine and tyramine are substitutes for the carrier. **(Ref. 1, p. 72; Ref. 4, p. 105; Ref. 12, p. 77)**

112. C. Nicotine, an alkaloid derived from plant sources, causes both acute and chronic toxicity. Its effects may vary considerably depending on the amount taken into the system. **(Ref. 1, p. 94; Ref. 2, p. 172; Ref. 3, p. 123; Ref. 4, pp. 180–183; Ref. 12, pp. 99–100)**

113. A. Norepinephrine is a potent stimulator of α_1-receptors, resulting in an increase in peripheral resistance and a reflex decrease in heart rate even though it is a β_1 stimulant. It has little effect on receptors mediating vasodilation. **(Ref. 1, p. 117; Ref. 2, pp. 121–122; Ref. 3, p. 145; Ref. 4, p. 193; Ref. 12, p. 124)**

114. B. Circulating epinephrine does not enter the central nervous system to any extent because it is a polar compound. It does have direct actions causing bronchial smooth muscle relaxation, mydriasis, hyperglycemia, and inhibition of the release of inflammatory mediators. (**Ref. 1,** pp. 115–117; **Ref. 2,** p. 124; **Ref. 3,** p. 147; **Ref. 4,** p. 196; **Ref. 12,** pp. 121–124)

115. E. Adrenergic receptor function can be modified by various adaptive changes including phosphorylation, internalization, and modification of portions of the signaling process. (**Ref. 1,** pp. 112–113; **Ref. 4,** pp. 112–113; **Ref. 12,** pp. 119–120)

116. C. The uterus is influenced by the hormonal background. Most adrenergic agents do not have much therapeutic usefulness with respect to uterine smooth muscle. The exception is β_2 agonists, which inhibit premature labor. (**Ref. 1,** pp. 116, 121; **Ref. 2,** p. 123; **Ref. 4,** p. 196; **Ref. 12,** pp. 123, 129)

117. A. The precursor to norepinephrine, dopamine, has effects that vary depending on the concentration employed. At low levels it dilates renal and intestinal vascular beds, but as concentrations increase it stimulates β_1-receptors markedly and causes intense α_1 activation. It does not readily cross the blood-brain barrier. (**Ref. 1,** p. 117; **Ref. 3,** p. 149; **Ref. 4,** p. 200; **Ref. 12,** pp. 124–125)

118. D. The oral use of β_2-adrenergic agonists has significant skeletal muscle tremor as a side effect. While it might be expected that tolerance and/or arrhythmias would occur, these are usually not a major clinical problem. Hyperglycemia is produced and insulin dosage may need to be adjusted. (**Ref. 1,** pp. 286, 287; **Ref. 4,** p. 206; **Ref. 12,** p. 136)

119. D. This derivative of atropine is administered by inhalation to treat asthma. Because of its polarity, it is a quaternary compound, and its actions tends to remain localized. As an anticholinergic, it causes dry mouth. (**Ref. 1,** p. 288; **Ref. 2,** p. 157; **Ref. 4,** pp. 159–160; **Ref. 12,** p. 315)

120. E. Metoprolol is a selective β_1-receptor antagonist and should not be confused with the β_2-selective agonist, metaproterenol. Beta agonists typically have an "-ol" ending, while antagonists have an "-olol" ending. (**Ref. 4,** pp. 191, 205, 234)

121. **A.** Agents that block the muscarinic receptor usually have widespread side effects and there has been an active search for selective agents, such as ipratropium and pirenzepine. Agents currently used cause cycloplegia and do not decrease gastric acid secretion unless high doses are employed. (**Ref. 1,** pp. 103, 104; **Ref. 2,** p. 153; **Ref. 4,** pp. 161–162; **Ref. 12,** p. 110)

122. **C.** There is the impression that *Amanita muscaria* poisoning results from excess acetylcholine. However, *A muscaria* also contains antimuscarinic alkaloids, which are responsible for its toxicity. *Amanita phalloides* is a form of poisoning that is slow in onset and often fatal. Pralidoxime is a quaternary compound that does not penetrate the CNS but can reverse organophosphate poisoning if the enzyme has not "aged." (**Ref. 1,** pp. 103, 104; **Ref. 4,** pp. 129, 141; **Ref. 12,** pp. 109–110)

123. **E.** By virtue of their structural chemistry, the quaternary amine, neostigmine, does not enter the CNS while the tertiary amine, physostigmine, does. They are both cholinesterase inhibitors. While the term "reversible" is a relative term, both of these compounds are relatively reversible when compared with organophosphate compounds. (**Ref. 1,** pp. 89–91; **Ref. 4,** p. 134; **Ref. 12,** pp. 94–95)

124. **C.** Acetylcholine, but not bethanechol, will be potentiated by pretreatment with a cholinesterase inhibitor because bethanechol is not a substrate. Hexamethonium, in contrast to decamethonium, blocks at ganglia. Scopolamine is a cholinergic muscarinic blocker. (**Ref. 1,** p. 91; **Ref. 4,** p. 126; **Ref. 12,** p. 97)

125. **B.** Pilocarpine is a naturally occurring cholinomimetic alkaloid that will activate muscarinic sites, inducing contraction of airways and the precipitation of an asthmatic episode. It is employed topically for open angle glaucoma, where it acts within minutes. (**Ref. 1,** pp. 92–94; **Ref. 2,** p. 149; **Ref. 3,** p. 106; **Ref. 4,** pp. 128–129; **Ref. 12,** pp. 98–99)

126. **B.** Cholinergic agonists delay AV conduction (increase conduction time) and inhibit the SA node. They would be additive with the indirect "vagal" effects of digitalis, and would have a negative inotropic action. (**Ref. 1,** pp. 86, 87; **Ref. 4,** p. 125; **Ref. 12,** pp. 92–93)

127. D. It is important to know the predominant tone at various effector sites when attempting to predict the action of a drug that blocks the ganglia. The iris is usually partially contracted. Blocking this effect leads to mydriasis. (**Ref. 1,** pp. 105, 106; **Ref. 2,** p. 174; **Ref. 3,** pp. 125, 126; **Ref. 4,** p. 183; **Ref. 12,** pp. 111, 112)

128. A. The belladonna alkaloids are competitive antagonists to the muscarinic actions of acetylcholine and can prevent the fall in blood pressure from a previously effective dose of acetylcholine. (**Ref. 1,** p. 101; **Ref. 4,** p. 155; **Ref. 12,** p. 105)

129. D. The α-adrenergic blocking drug phentolamine competitively antagonizes the blood pressure rise caused by the nicotinic action of the larger dose of acetylcholine. Ephedrine, epinephrine or phenylephrine would increase blood pressure while phentolamine would cause a sustained decrease. This nicotinic action results in epinephrine release from the adrenal gland plus norepinephrine release due to sympathetic ganglionic stimulation. (**Ref. 4,** p. 124)

130. C. The increased blood pressure resulting from epinephrine administration is shorter in duration than with ephedrine or phenylephrine. With epinephrine, the heart rate is usually increased unless the dose is very large; with phenylephrine, reflex bradycardia occurs because it stimulates only α-adrenergic receptors. (**Ref. 1,** pp. 117, 118; **Ref. 2,** pp. 126, 127; **Ref. 4,** pp. 192, 207; **Ref. 12,** pp. 124–125)

131. D. Phentolamine is an equilibrium-competitive α-adrenergic antagonist, with a quicker and shorter duration of action than the haloalkylamines. The immediate effect of slow intravenous administration is reduced vasoconstriction and some fall in blood pressure; repeating the administration of epinephrine elicits only β-adrenergic effects. (**Ref. 1,** p. 126; **Ref. 3,** p. 160; **Ref. 4,** p. 223; **Ref. 12,** pp. 134)

132. C. While phenoxybenzamine is a nonequilibrium α-adrenergic blocking agent it will also block muscarinic, histaminic, and serotonergic receptors. These other receptors are inhibited at higher doses of phenoxybenzamine. The α-adrenergic blocker may be long lasting since it is dependent on synthesis of new receptors. (**Ref. 1,** p. 127; **Ref. 2,** p. 132; **Ref. 4,** pp. 221, 224; **Ref. 12,** p. 135)

133. **E.** Yohimbine is an alkaloid that is of interest because of its specific α_2-adrenergic–blocking activity. It has received new interest in treating male sexual dysfunction, but it is difficult to document whether this is a true pharmacologic effect or simply useful for psychologic impotence. (**Ref. 1,** p. 127; **Ref. 4,** pp. 221, 229; **Ref. 12,** p. 135)

134. **B.** The discovery of the α_1 and α_2 subtypes of adrenergic receptors has led to the development of specific antagonists and revitalized the use of α-blockers for the treatment of hypertension. Since α_2 receptors are not blocked, these agents lessen the incidence of tachycardia. However, they are known to cause marked hypertension as a first dose phenomenon. (**Ref. 1,** p. 151; **Ref. 2,** p. 135; **Ref. 3,** p. 162; **Ref. 4,** pp. 221, 226, 227; **Ref. 12,** p. 159)

135. **E.** Propranolol and pindolol are both nonselective but only pindolol stimulates receptors and may be preferred in patients with limited cardiac function. (**Ref. 1,** p. 132; **Ref. 4,** pp. 229, 235; **Ref. 12,** pp. 141, 158)

136. **A.** Propranolol in high concentrations will stabilize membranes (quinidine-like effect). The clinical significance of this effect is not known since the antiarrhythmic action is related to β-blocking activity. (**Ref. 1,** p. 132; **Ref. 2,** p. 138; **Ref. 3,** p. 164; **Ref. 4,** p. 231; **Ref. 12,** p. 140)

137. **B.** Haloperidol is a selective D_2-receptor blocker in the renal vascular beds. (**Ref. 1,** p. 398; **Ref. 4,** pp. 260–261; **Ref. 12,** p. 435)

138. **D.** Ergonovine, one of the ergot alkaloids, is useful in treatment of postpartum hemorrhage. Ergotamine has been employed for migraine headaches. Ergot alkaloids have a complex pattern of action. They are adrenergic-blocking agents, partial serotonin agonists, and they cause intense contraction of smooth muscles (vascular and uterine). (**Ref. 1,** pp. 125, 246; **Ref. 3,** p. 162; **Ref. 4,** p. 228; **Ref. 12,** pp. 270–271)

139. A. Propranolol and other certain β-adrenergic blockers, have been shown to be effective, if given after a myocardial infarction, in improving mortality statistics and in preventing recurrence by a mechanism that is not understood. (**Ref. 1**, p. 114; **Ref. 3**, p. 165; **Ref. 4**, p. 240; **Ref. 6**, p. 551; **Ref. 12**, p. 142)

140. A. Ganglionic blocking agents inhibit acetylcholine at nicotinic ganglionic sites. They have ganglionic selectivity but are nonselective because they inhibit both sympathetic and parasympathetic ganglia. Trimetaphan is a ganglionic blocking agent with a short duration of action that is used to produce controlled hypotension. (**Ref. 1**, p. 106; **Ref. 2**, p. 175; **Ref. 3**, pp. 124–125; **Ref. 4**, p. 184; **Ref. 12**, pp. 111–112)

141. D. Tyrosine hydroxylase, located in the neuronal side of the adrenergic neuron, is inhibited by metyrosine. This is the rate-limiting step in catecholamine biosynthesis. Metyrosine is used in the treatment of pheochromocytoma. (**Ref. 1**, p. 128; **Ref. 2**, p. 244; **Ref. 3**, p. 171; **Ref. 4**, p. 796; **Ref. 12**, pp. 136–137)

142. B. Selective β_1-receptor antagonism of a competitive nature is produced by metoprolol. β-blockers are identified by the -olol ending. Metoprolol has no partial agonist activity. (**Ref. 1**, p. 132; **Ref. 2**, pp. 137–139; **Ref. 3**, p. 166; **Ref. 4**, p. 236; **Ref. 12**, pp. 140–141)

143. D. The compound bretylium has local anesthetic activity. It accumulates in adrenergic nerve endings, releases catecholamines, and then prevents the release of norepinephrine. It is used in life-threatening cardiac arrhythmias, not as a first-line agent. (**Ref. 1**, p. 206; **Ref. 2**, pp. 303, 304; **Ref. 3**, p. 169; **Ref. 4**, p. 866; **Ref. 12**, pp. 222–223)

144. B. Compounds that interfere with the uptake mechanism responsible for terminating the response to catecholamines potentiate exogenously administered amines. They also inhibit the action of indirectly-acting amines, such as tyramine. Tranylcypromine would also potentiate the response by inhibiting metabolism by MAO, but it is not a local anesthetic. (**Ref. 1**, pp. 79, 119; **Ref. 2**, p. 366; **Ref. 3**, pp. 92, 95; **Ref. 4**, p. 116; **Ref. 12**, pp. 84–126)

145. A. Cholinesterase inhibitors are considered indirect-acting cholinomimetics. These agents do not stimulate receptors in clinically used doses. They are effective due to the accumulation of acetylcholine at nicotinic and muscarinic sites. It is muscarinic activation that causes salivation. Since these compounds are not selective, this increased salivation may be bothersome. (**Ref. 1**, p. 94; **Ref. 2**, p. 164; **Ref. 3**, pp. 108, 109; **Ref. 12**, p. 100)

146. D. Propranolol administration will result in an increased sensitivity to adrenergic amines. This is due to receptor up-regulation. The drug must be removed slowly, over one to two weeks, to allow the body to readjust. Pindolol has intrinsic sympathomimetic activity that is reported to lessen supersensitivity responses; however caution should be exercised in withdrawing patients from this drug. (**Ref. 1**, p. 136; **Ref. 3**, p. 165; **Ref. 12**, p. 145)

147. B. The blood pressure responses show essentially no change in the response to vagal stimulation or acetylcholine. The β_1 cardiac component and the β_2 vasodilatory component of the blood pressure trace are missing after epinephrine. Norepinephrine does not stimulate β_2 receptors; however, the β_1 cardiac response is eliminated. This pattern would be observed after nonselective β-adrenergic blockade. (**Ref. 1**, p. 117; **Ref. 2**, p. 112; **Ref. 3**, p. 162; **Ref. 4**, p. 231; **Ref. 12**, pp. 122–123)

148. C. The effects of acetylcholine, whether released by vagal nerve stimulation or administered exogenously, would be potentiated. Vagal escape might well be observed. The responses to epinephrine and norepinephrine would be unchanged. Only the responses on blood pressure due to actions on the heart and blood vessels are shown by these traces. (**Ref. 1**, p. 91; **Ref. 2**, p. 164; **Ref. 4**, p. 138; **Ref. 12**, p. 97)

149. A. Epinephrine is a nonselective stimulator of both α and β receptors. Norepinephrine action is exhibited by choice B since it has minimal activity at β_2 receptors. Isoproterenol exhibits nonselective β receptor activity, choice E. Patterns C and D are characteristic of antagonists, C of a nonselective α antagonist and D of labetalol. (**Ref. 1**, pp. 110, 125, 133; **Ref. 3**, p. 143; **Ref. 4**, pp. 192, 225, 228; **Ref. 12**, pp. 117, 134)

150. **C.** Both norepinephrine and dopamine activate cardiac (β_1) adrenoreceptors. Phenylephrine has β activity only at high concentrations, it is used as an α_1 agonist. Phentolamine and propranolol are nonselective blockers of α and β receptors, respectively. (**Ref. 1,** pp. 110; **Ref. 2,** pp. 122, 126; **Ref. 4,** pp. 198, 200, 206; **Ref. 12,** p. 117)

151. **D.** Catecholamines are stored in granules in adrenergic nerve endings; this source of catecholamines is depleted by reserpine. Norepinephrine, a direct acting agent, is not stored extraneuronally, is potentiated by tricyclic antidepressants, and is not inhibited by indirectly-acting amines. Indirectly-acting amines release norepinephrine from a small cytoplasmic storage pool. (**Ref. 1,** pp. 72, 73; **Ref. 3,** pp. 95, 150; **Ref. 4,** p. 105; **Ref. 12,** p. 77)

152. **D.** Methacholine has selectivity for muscarinic versus nicotinic receptors and is hydrolyzed at a slower rate by acetylcholinesterase than acetylcholine. It is resistant to nonspecific cholinesterase. (**Ref. 1,** p. 84; **Ref. 3,** p. 103; **Ref. 4,** p. 123; **Ref. 12,** p. 91)

153. **B.** The primary action of carbachol is on the intestine and on the urinary bladder. It penetrates to nicotinic sites. This includes all ganglia, skeletal muscle, and the adrenal medulla. (**Ref. 2,** p. 148; **Ref. 4,** p. 124)

154. **A.** Because acetylcholine is so rapidly hydrolyzed, the neurotransmitter has virtually no therapeutic use. Derivatives that have resistance to enzymatic degradation have been synthesized to provide longer duration of action and some selectivity at organ sites. (**Ref. 1,** p. 84; **Ref. 2,** p. 146; **Ref. 3,** p. 103; **Ref. 4,** p. 122; **Ref. 12,** p. 90)

155. **A.** Agents that activate the muscarinic receptor may produce untoward effects in patients with underlying conditions. In asthmatics they cause bronchial smooth-muscle contraction. In patients with angina pectoris, the danger is a hypotensive response that may reduce coronary blood flow. In patients with gastric ulcer, the stimulation of gastric acid secretion would be undesirable. (**Ref. 1,** p. 94; **Ref. 2,** p. 148; **Ref. 3,** p. 104; **Ref. 4,** p. 126)

156. B. Intoxication with atropine also includes a rapid/weak pulse, flushed skin (scarlet color), widely dilated pupils, and ataxia. This alkaloid produces both peripheral cholinergic blockage and central nervous system effects. (**Ref. 1,** p. 104; **Ref. 2,** p. 158; **Ref. 3,** pp. 117, 119; **Ref. 4,** p. 158; **Ref. 12,** p. 110)

157. D. Ganglionic stimulants such as nicotine do not show specificity for nicotine receptors. The effects observed are unpredictable, since nicotine has low selectivity at nicotinic sites and it first stimulates then blocks receptors. The major interest in nicotine was related to its acute and chronic toxicity. However, the use of nicotine patches has led to investigation of this compound in other disease states. (**Ref. 1,** p. 94; **Ref. 2,** p. 172; **Ref. 3,** p. 123; **Ref. 4,** p. 180; **Ref. 12,** pp. 99–100)

158. E. Propranolol is a nonselective β-adrenergic antagonist. It is competitive in action and is frequently effective in preventing, but not relieving, migraine headaches. The mechanism of this effect is not known. (**Ref. 1,** pp. 134, 135; **Ref. 2,** p. 141; **Ref. 3,** p. 165; **Ref. 4,** p. 946; **Ref. 12,** p. 143)

159. A. Cromolyn is administered by metered-dose inhaler or by nebulizer inhalation. It inhibits antigen-induced liberation of histamine and leukotrienes. The compound does not relax bronchial smooth muscle, nor does it block combination of histamine or other substances with the receptor. (**Ref. 1,** p. 281; **Ref. 2,** p. 519; **Ref. 3,** p. 504; **Ref. 4,** p. 631; **Ref. 12,** pp. 308–309)

160. B. Minoxidil is an arteriolar vasodilator with little effect on capacitance vessels. It causes salt and water retention, cardiac stimulation, and excessive hair growth, hence its use for male pattern baldness (topical application). In order to reduce the dose and toxicity of minoxidil, a diuretic and a β-adrenergic blocking drug can be administered with minoxidil. It is reserved for severe hypertension. (**Ref. 1,** p. 153; **Ref. 2,** p. 234; **Ref. 3,** pp. 176, 177; **Ref. 4,** pp. 801–803; **Ref. 6,** pp. 796–797; **Ref. 12,** p. 161)

161. C. Timolol is effective topically in the treatment of chronic wide-angle glaucoma. It decreases the production of aqueous humor. Timolol is a β-adrenergic antagonist, metoprolol is β_1 selective. Other β-blockers will also reduce intraocular pressure; however, timolol has been preferred because it lacks a local anesthetic effect. **(Ref. 1,** p. 134; **Ref. 2,** p. 140; **Ref. 3,** p. 166; **Ref. 8,** pp. 236, 240; **Ref. 12,** p. 141)

162. **A.** Pilocarpine has been used for many years in the treatment of chronic simple and secondary glaucoma. It is an alkaloid with muscarinic actions; its actions are similar but more prolonged than those of acetylcholine. **(Ref. 1,** p. 92; **Ref. 2,** p. 167; **Ref. 4,** p. 129; **Ref. 12,** p. 98)

163. **E.** Clonidine initially causes some stimulation of postsynaptic peripheral α_2-adrenergic receptors. However, when it is administered orally in small doses, any initial rise in blood pressure is minimal or absent. **(Ref. 1,** pp. 145, 146; **Ref. 2,** p.246; **Ref. 3,** p.183; **Ref. 4,** p. 208; **Ref. 12,** pp. 153, 154)

164. **C.** Amphetamines suppress feeding and cause weight loss by decreasing food intake; however, this effect is not sustained because of the rapid development of tolerance in humans. There is no major effect on metabolism. Amphetamine is no longer recommended for treatment of obesity, and this use is illegal in many if not all states. **(Ref. 1,** p. 121; **Ref. 2,** p. 128; **Ref. 3,** p. 155; **Ref. 4,** p. 211; **Ref. 12,** p. 129)

165. **B.** Receptor subtypes have been identified in tissues. The blockade or the stimulation of receptor subtypes results in greater selectivity of action. While α_2-receptors are located both pre- and postsynaptically, a major consequence of blocking α_2-receptors is an increased catecholamine outflow. The inhibition process is inhibited. **(Ref. 1,** p. 75; **Ref. 2,** p. 131; **Ref. 3,** p. 142; **Ref. 4,** p. 103; **Ref. 12,** pp. 78, 79)

166. **C.** Propranolol is the β-adrenergic blocker against which others are compared. It causes receptor upregulation, requiring slow withdrawal. It is nonselective, does not block α-receptors, and does undergo first-pass metabolism. It has considerable membrane stabilization activity, and local anesthetic effect; however, its antiarrhythmic action is thought to be due to β-adrenergic receptor blockade. **(Ref. 1,** pp. 131, 132; **Ref. 2,** p. 139; **Ref. 3,** pp. 166, 167; **Ref. 4,** pp. 232–234; **Ref. 12,** pp. 140–141)

167. D. Muscarinic receptor activation will cause all of the actions listed except inhibition of endothelial dependent relaxing factor (EDRF). It is the release of this substance that is responsible for the vasodilation induced by cholinomimetics. (**Ref. 1,** pp. 86, 87; **Ref. 2,** pp. 146, 147, 151; **Ref. 4,** p. 124; **Ref. 12,** pp. 92–93)

168. C. Neostigmine is considered a reversible inhibitor of acetylcholinesterase even though it covalently binds to the enzyme. Neostigmine and physostigmine carbamylate the enzyme. The organophosphates phosphorylate it. (**Ref. 1,** pp. 90, 91; **Ref. 2,** p. 163; **Ref. 3,** pp. 110–112; **Ref. 4,** pp. 133–135; **Ref. 12,** p. 94)

4

Drugs Affecting the Cardiovascular System

DIRECTIONS (Questions 169–196): Each of the questions or incomplete statements below is followed by five suggested answers or completions. Select the **one** that is best in each case.

169. The preferred agent for hypertensive emergencies is
   A. diazoxide
   B. sodium nitroprusside
   C. propranolol
   D. captopril
   E. clonidine

170. All of the following statements about nitroglycerin are true EXCEPT
   A. nitrates relax the smooth muscles of both arteries and veins
   B. low levels of nitroglycerin cause a greater venodilation than arterial dilation
   C. the primary action of nitroglycerin is to increase coronary blood flow
   D. nitrates appear to cause a redistribution of coronary blood flow
   E. nitroglycerin has a greater relaxant effect on large versus small coronary arteries

171. Digoxin would be the choice for long-term treatment of congestive heart failure resulting from
   A. essential hypertension
   B. thyrotoxicosis
   C. severe myocardial infarction
   D. anemia
   E. mechanical obstruction

172. The effects of quinidine include
   A. an increase in the force of myocardial contraction
   B. an indirect effect to decrease atrial-ventricular (AV) conduction time
   C. vasoconstriction
   D. activation of sodium channels
   E. hypertensive episodes

173. Which of the following statements are true regarding the diagrams in Figure 4?
   A. The action of class I antiarrhythmic drugs should be diagrammed as the change occurring between panels B and D
   B. Digitalis would be expected to suppress the type of activity diagrammed in panel A and convert it to panel C-type response
   C. The monophasic action potential shown in panel E could be converted by procainamide to the pattern seen in panel A
   D. Calcium channel blockers act primarily to alter the phase 4 potential shown in panel E
   E. Verapamil restores and stimulates the delayed depolarization diagrammed in panel C

174. Which panel in Figure 4, depicts the phenomenon of early after-depolarization?

175. All of the following are considered mechanisms of antiarrhythmic drug action EXCEPT
   A. calcium channel blockade
   B. inhibition of catecholamine action on the heart
   C. sodium channel blockade
   D. increasing the rate of dV/dt in phase 4
   E. prolongation of the effective refractory period

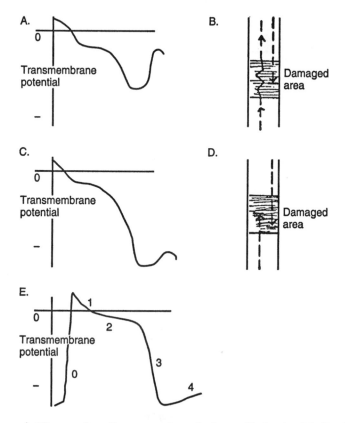

Figure 4 (Composite diagram adapted from Goth A: *Medical Pharmacology,* 11th Ed. St. Louis, CV Mosby, 1984, p. 439; Gilman AG, Goodman LS, Rall TW, Murad F: *Goodman and Gilman's The Pharmacological Basis of Therapeutics,* 7th Ed. New York, Macmillan, 1985, pp. 752–753, with permission.)

176. In the therapy of congestive heart failure, the most important pharmacologic action of digitalis is its ability to
  A. produce diuresis in edematous patients
  B. reduce venous pressure
  C. increase myocardial contractile force
  D. increase heart rate
  E. decrease pacemaker automaticity in cells of the bundle of His

177. Of the following cardiac glycosides, which has the clearly superior (larger) therapeutic index?
A. Ouabain
B. Digoxin
C. Digitoxin
D. Deslanoside
E. None of the above is superior to the others

178. Digoxin differs from digitoxin in that digoxin
A. has a longer half-life
B. is completely absorbed from the gastrointestinal tract
C. has a half-life that is dependent on renal function
D. is bound extensively to plasma proteins
E. is metabolized extensively by the liver

179. When digitalis is given to the typical patient with congestive failure and atrial fibrillation
A. cardiac output is unchanged
B. ventricular rate is slowed by both vagal and direct effects
C. ventricular efficiency is decreased
D. a decrease in heart rate is a primary effect
E. none of the above occurs

180. Which of the following statements regarding blood lipids is true?
A. No convincing data have been published yet to show a high correlation between patients with familial hypercholesterolemia and myocardial infarction
B. Epinephrine can cause a rise in serum lipids, but chronic administration has no effect on experimental atherosclerosis
C. Polyunsaturated oils, such as corn oil, will promote fecal excretion of cholesterol
D. In patients, clofibrate is more effective in lowering plasma triglycerides than plasma cholesterol
E. Although there are several patterns of hyperlipoproteinemia, therapy is the same for all types

181. Which of the following statements is true concerning cholestyra-mine?
    A. It inhibits free fatty-acid release from adipose tissue
    B. It releases lipoprotein lipase
    C. It is an anion-exchange resin that binds bile acid in the human intestinal lumen
    D. It blocks the final step in the formation of cholesterol in the body
    E. When used in large doses, it decreases serum cholesterol, triglycerides, and phospholipids, possibly via an effect on synthesis

182. Quinidine is either contraindicated or should be used with caution in all of the following EXCEPT
    A. complete AV block
    B. digitalis intoxication
    C. severe congestive heart failure
    D. atrial fibrillation of recent origin
    E. a history of thrombocytopenic purpura due to previous use of quinidine

183. The syndrome of cinchonism includes all of the following symp-toms EXCEPT
    A. tinnitus
    B. delirium
    C. disturbed vision
    D. hypertensive reaction
    E. headache

184. Side effects that might be expected with hydralazine include all of the following EXCEPT
    A. headache
    B. palpitations
    C. AV block
    D. anginal attacks
    E. acute rheumatoid symptoms

185. Regarding the effects of digitalis on conduction and refractory period, all of the following statements are true EXCEPT
    A. AV nodal conduction is slowed by the vagal effect, but this is opposed by the direct effect

B. the P-R interval of the ECG is prolonged
C. the refractory period of the AV node is prolonged
D. the refractory period of the ventricle is usually either unchanged or shortened
E. the refractory period of the atrium is usually shortened in humans

186. In the typical patient with congestive heart failure, digitalis would be expected to do all of the following EXCEPT
A. decrease the diastolic heart size
B. increase the cardiac output
C. increase sympathetic activity
D. increase vital capacity
E. decrease blood volume

187. The antihypertensive agent that acts by inhibiting the formation of angiotensin is
A. hydralazine
B. captopril
C. minoxidil
D. propranolol
E. prazosin

188. The effects of digoxin on transmembrane electrograms would be expected to include
A. a decrease in the rate of change of dV/dt in phase 4
B. a lengthening of phase 2 and 3
C. the production of early after-depolarizations
D. an increase in the slope of phase 4
E. an increase in action potential duration

189. Increased contractile force development after digoxin administration
A. is qualitatively different from that of digitoxin
B. depends on the stimulation of Na^+, K^+-ATPase
C. is due to inhibition of sodium transport
D. results in increased intracellular sodium, which exchanges for calcium
E. depends on increased levels of intracellular ATP

190. Antiarrhythmic agents would decrease generation arrhythmias by
   A. increasing dV/dt in phase 0
   B. decreasing resting membrane potential
   C. converting unidirectional conduction to bidirectional block
   D. altering threshold potential
   E. lengthening refractory period

191. In reference to antiarrhythmic drugs, all the following statements are true EXCEPT
   A. class I_c agents are arrhythmogenic
   B. encainide has been demonstrated to increase the risk of sudden cardiac death
   C. flecainide will effectively prevent unsustained ventricular arrhythmias in patients with a recent myocardial infarction
   D. cimetidine may cause an increase in toxicity of encainide
   E. propafenone may cause a systemic lupus erythematosus (SLE)-like syndrome

192. All of the following statements are true EXCEPT
   A. heparin acts both in vitro and in vivo
   B. coumadin acts in vivo only
   C. heparin may enter the placenta causing internal bleeding
   D. coumadin is considered a vitamin K antagonist
   E. heparin must be administered parenterally

193. The lowering of plasma lipids by lovastatin occurs because it
   A. inhibits HMG coenzyme A (CoA) reductase
   B. binds bile acids
   C. it inhibits VLDL secretion
   D. stimulates HMG CoA excretion
   E. increases the activity of lipoprotein lipase

194. In the reduction of elevated blood pressure all of the following pairings are appropriate EXCEPT
   A. enalapril/acetylcholinesterase inhibitor
   B. methyldopa/α_2-agonist
   C. metyrosine/tyrosine hydroxylase inhibitor
   D. clonidine/α_2-agonist
   E. prazosin/α_1-antagonist

195. Organic nitrates
 A. stimulate cAMP production
 B. inhibit the synthesis of cGMP
 C. result in the formation of NO
 D. block cGMP-dependent protein kinase
 E. lead to phosphorylation of myosin light chain kinase

196. All the following statements are true regarding procainamide EXCEPT
 A. replacement of the nitrogen with a carbon results in procaine
 B. N-acetylprocainamide, a metabolite, has antiarrhythmic action
 C. Procainamide may produce thrombocytopenia
 D. an SLE-like syndrome is apt to occur sooner in "slow acetylators" of procainamide
 E. procainamide can cause profound decrease in blood pressure

---

DIRECTIONS (Questions 197–202): This section consists of two clinical situations followed by a series of questions. Study the situations and select the **one** best answer to each question following them.

Questions 197–199: A patient appears in the emergency room with an accelerated ventricular heart rate approaching 190 beats/min. Upon discussion with the spouse, it is determined that the patient is taking digoxin along with hydrochlorothiazide and eats large quantities of bananas.

197. The first action taken should be
 A. administration of quinidine
 B. intravenous lidocaine
 C. intravenous potassium
 D. oral procainamide
 E. intravenous drip of magnesium

198. An important element in the treatment of digitalis intoxication that is often overlooked is
 A. administration of Fab antibody fragments
 B. monitoring the electrocardiogram
 C. determination of serum potassium levels
 D. withdrawal of the cardiac glycoside
 E. administration of potassium

199. In the above case, the first step should not be administration of potassium ion because
  A. it could lead to cardiac arrest
  B. potassium is difficult to administer
  C. magnesium is a better choice
  D. automaticity may be increased
  E. AV block may occur

Questions 200–202: Early in September, a female patient arrives at your office complaining of shortness of breath and pounding in the chest. On examination you find that her blood pressure is 140/90, heart rate is 120 beats/min, and no "P" waves are present in the ECG.

200. The decision is to administer digitalis because
  A. congestive heart failure is suspected
  B. it will dilate the airways and improve breathing
  C. the "P" waves need to be restored
  D. the patient has hypertension
  E. cardiac glycosides have minimal effects on the ECG

201. The safest approach to therapy is
  A. digitalization with digoxin
  B. digitalization with digitoxin
  C. intravenous administration of acetyl strophanthidin
  D. administration of maintenance doses of digoxin
  E. administration of maintenance doses of digitoxin

202. The earliest sign of effectiveness would probably be
  A. diuresis
  B. a decrease in heart rate
  C. yellow-green vision
  D. gynecomastia
  E. diarrhea

DIRECTIONS (Questions 203–206): Each group of questions below consists of five lettered headings followed by a list of numbered words, phrases, or statements. For each numbered word, phrase, or statement, select the **one** lettered heading that is most closely associated with it. Each lettered heading may be selected once, more than once, or not at all.

Questions 203–206:
   A. Phenytoin
   B. Papaverine
   C. Digitalis
   D. Adenosine
   E. Propranolol

203. When used as an antagonist to digitalis-induced arrhythmias, can increase the degree of AV block

204. A drug that is most useful in treating digitalis-induced supraventricular and ventricular ectopic rhythms

205. Effective in heart failure associated with low cardiac output

206. Short-acting agent useful for termination of supraventricular tachycardia

Questions 207–209:
   A. Digoxin
   B. Cholestyramine
   C. Digitoxin
   D. Quinidine
   E. Nitroglycerin

207. Cardiac glycoside that undergoes extensive hepatic degradation

208. Inhibits vitamin K absorption

209. Increases conductivity of AV node by blocking the vagus

Questions 210–211:
   A. Amrinone
   B. Amiodarone
   C. Disopyramide
   D. Labetalol
   E. Bretylium

210. A positive cardiac inotropic agent

211. An antiarrhythmic agent originally developed for angina

212. This antihypertensive compound will inhibit both α_1- and β-receptor function

Questions 213–216:
   A. Lidocaine
   B. Quinidine
   C. Tocainide
   D. Bretylium
   E. Propranolol

213. Major adverse reactions include tremor and gastrointestinal upset

214. Bound to α_1-acid glycoprotein

215. Often administered with a preservative or vasoconstrictor

216. Only effective when administered intravenously

Questions 217–220:
   A. Digoxin
   B. Quinidine
   C. Heparin
   D. Dicumarol
   E. Lidocaine

217. Antagonized by protamine

218. Electrocardiographic changes in lead 1 produced by this drug (changes are shown in Figure 5)

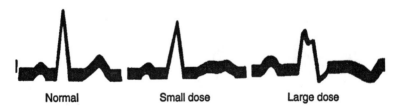

Normal   Small dose   Large dose

Figure 5 (Adapted from Burch GE, Winsor T: *A Primer of Electrocardiography.* Philadelphia, Lea and Febiger, 1960, with permission.)

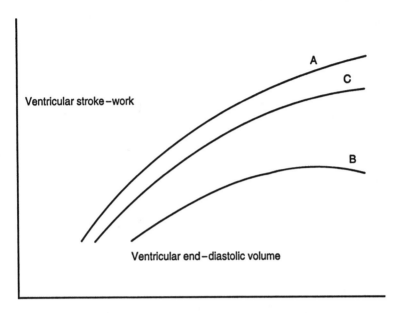

Figure 6

219. Drug responsible for the change from curve B to curve C in this graph of ventricular end-diastolic volume on the abscissa and ventricular stroke-work on the ordinate where A is normal, B is cardiac failure, and C is cardiac failure after treatment with one of the drugs (Figure 6)

220. In Figure 6, a drug that could cause a shift from curve A to curve B

DIRECTIONS (Questions 221–228): Each of the questions or incomplete statements below is followed by five suggested answers or completions. Select the **one** that is best in each case.

221. In comparing calcium channel blockers
  A. nifedipine produces marked vasodilation
  B. calcium channel blockers are very effective for ventricular arrhythmias
  C. verapamil decreases blood flow in skeletal muscle vascular beds
  D. diltiazem increases coronary vascular resistance
  E. verapamil produces minimal inhibition of AV conduction

222. Side effects common to calcium channel blockers include all of the following EXCEPT
   A. dizziness and flushing
   B. worsening of myocardial ischemia
   C. tachycardia
   D. excessive vasodilation
   E. diarrhea

223. Minoxidil
   A. causes venovasodilation
   B. stimulates diuresis
   C. may cause a marked decrease in heart rate
   D. stimulates the growth of hair
   E. is only effective intravenously or topically

224. The management of angina pectoris includes all of the following EXCEPT
   A. organic nitrites
   B. calcium channel blockers
   C. β-adrenergic antagonists
   D. organic nitrates
   E. inhibitors of platelet aggregation

225. Effective administration routes of nitroglycerin for angina pectoris include all of the following EXCEPT
   A. transdermal
   B. ointment
   C. sublingual
   D. intravenous
   E. oral

226. The use of vasodilators in the treatment of congestive heart failure is based on
   A. the predominant effect of these compounds on venous smooth muscle
   B. an effect of nitroprusside to inhibit cyclic-GMP formation
   C. the development of additional contractile force in the heart
   D. the reduction of cardiac preload and/or afterload
   E. an increase in contractile force development

227. Electrocardiographic effects of digitalis include all of the following EXCEPT
   A. lengthening of the P-R interval
   B. shortening of the Q-T interval
   C. inversion of the T wave
   D. widening of the QRS complex in Wolf-Parkinson-White (WPW) syndrome
   E. widening of the QRS complex in most patients.

228. Regarding the cardiac glycosides
   A. the aglycon is devoid of action on the heart
   B. the compound possesses sugar molecules as part of its structure
   C. a carboxyl group at position 17 is required for optimal activity
   D. the unsaturated lactone is an essential component of its structure
   E. the hydroxyl group at position 14 is necessary for biologic activity

229. Treatment of arrhythmias
   A. should involve lidocaine as a first choice drug in most situations
   B. has little danger when compared with other types of drug therapy
   C. requires accurate identification of the type of arrhythmia, generation or conduction
   D. requires serious consideration of non-drug therapy
   E. is uncomplicated when compared with other types of drug therapy

---

DIRECTIONS (Questions 230–237): Each group of questions below consists of five lettered headings followed by a list of numbered words, phrases, or statements. For each numbered word, phrase, or statement, select the **one** lettered heading that is most closely associated with it. Each lettered heading may be selected once, more than once, or not at all.

Questions 230–233:
   A. Amiodarone
   B. Propranolol
   C. Quinidine
   D. Verapamil
   E. Lidocaine

230. This compound possesses both atropine-like activity and oxytocic activity

231. Prolongation of the duration of the action potential is a unique feature

232. Agent to be selected for management of paroxysmal supraventricular arrhythmia in an individual who engages in regular exercise such as jogging

233. Shortens the action potential duration in Purkinje fibers

Questions 234–237:
- **A.** Metyrosine
- **B.** Clonidine
- **C.** Prazosin
- **D.** Trimetaphan
- **E.** Guanethidine

234. A centrally-acting antihypertensive agent

235. Acts to inhibit the rate-limiting step in catecholamine biosynthesis

236. Administered intravenously to produce short periods of hypotension

237. This compound is ineffective in the presence of uptake inhibitors

238. In the treatment of angina pectoris
- **A.** β-adrenergic antagonists provide effective vasodilation
- **B.** propranolol is the only β-blocker that is therapeutically effective
- **C.** β-adrenergic blocking agents are most effective in vasospastic angina
- **D.** β-adrenergic blocker withdrawal may cause myocardial infarction
- **E.** the combination of organic nitrates and β-blockers are contraindicated

239. All of the following are true regarding disturbances in cardiac rhythm EXCEPT
- **A.** abnormal rhythm may be due to a defect in conduction
- **B.** arrhythmias may occur due to ectopic pacemakers

C. an increase in spontaneous depolarization of cardiac tissue increases heart rate
D. inhibition of AV conduction may protect the ventricle
E. unidirectional conduction can be improved by administering catecholamines

240. The use of ACE inhibitors is contraindicated in
A. asthma
B. hyperlipidemia
C. bilateral renal artery stenosis
D. decreased renal function
E. diabetes mellitus

241. Which of the following pharmacological agents alter plasminogen after binding to fibrin?
A. Streptokinase
B. Urokinase
C. Tissue-plasminogen activator
D. α_2-Antiplasmin
E. Aminocaproic acid

242. The major untoward effect of heparin is
A. bleeding
B. crossing the placenta
C. elevation of hepatic transaminases
D. allergic reactions
E. inhibition of aldosterone synthesis

243. All of the following are drug interactions involving quinidine EXCEPT
A. cimetidine stimulates the hepatic metabolism of quinidine
B. phenytoin and the barbiturates stimulate the metabolism of quinidine
C. digoxin levels may increase if quinidine is administered
D. antacids may lead to elevations in quinidine levels
E. acetazolamide may increase the plasma concentration of quinidine

244. The toxicity of most antiarrhythmic agents has led to concerted efforts to produce compounds similar to lidocaine but which have oral effectiveness. A congener of lidocaine that is orally effective is
   A. procainamide
   B. tocainide
   C. disopyramide
   D. amiodarone
   E. esmolol

245. Niacin or nicotinic acid
   A. inhibits HMG-CoA reductase
   B. increases plasma levels of VLDL
   C. lowers triglycerides due to its action as a vitamin
   D. should not be combined with a bile acid-binding resin
   E. inhibits the production of VLDL in the liver

246. Procainamide
   A. causes thrombocytopenia as a major side effect
   B. produces cardiac stimulation
   C. may cause an SLE-like syndrome
   D. rarely produces antinuclear antibodies
   E. has a hypertensive action

247. All of the following are extracardiac effects of digoxin EXCEPT
   A. yellow-green vision
   B. hallucinations
   C. diarrhea
   D. reduction in breast size
   E. cardiac arrhythmias

248. Urokinase
   A. directly activates plasminogen
   B. activates plasminogen after urokinase binds to plasminogen
   C. must bind to fibrin before plasminogen is activated
   D. activity depends on the level of calcium present
   E. is produced from streptokinase

DIRECTIONS (Questions 249–253): Each group of questions below consists of five lettered headings followed by a list of numbered words, phrases, or statements. For each numbered word, phrase, or statement, select the **one** lettered heading that is most closely associated with it. Each lettered heading may be selected once, more than once, or not at all.

    A. Warfarin
    B. Heparin
    C. Vitamin K
    D. Saralasin
    E. Spironolactone

249. Has an antilipemic effect

250. Antagonist of angiotensin

251. Antagonizes the action of oral anticoagulants

252. Aldosterone antagonist

253. Potassium-sparing diuretic

Drugs Affecting the Cardiovascular System

Answers and Discussion

169. **B.** Intravenous administration of sodium nitroprusside will cause rapid vasodilation of arterial and venous vessels. Diazoxide is not useful for all types of emergencies. The other agents are used orally for long-term management. (**Ref. 1,** p. 159; **Ref. 2,** pp. 235, 236; **Ref. 3,** p. 177; **Ref. 4,** p. 804; **Ref. 9,** p. 280; **Ref. 12,** pp. 161, 167)

170. **C.** The beneficial effect of nitroglycerin is not fully understood, but it appears that it increases oxygen supply to the myocardium and, probably most importantly, decreases cardiac work, thus reducing oxygen demand. (**Ref. 1,** pp. 165, 166; **Ref. 3,** p. 442; **Ref. 4,** p. 766; **Ref. 12,** p. 172)

171. **A.** The most common precipitating cause of congestive heart failure is essential hypertension, where cardiac output is low. The other four precipitating factors are not effectively managed with cardiac glycosides. (**Ref. 1,** pp. 184, 185; **Ref. 4,** pp. 830, 831; **Ref. 12,** pp. 197–198)

172. **B.** Quinidine is a blocker of sodium channels, resulting in negative inotropic effects. It also causes vasodilation and may cause hypotensive (quinidine syncope) episodes. Because of its anti-

cholinergic effect, AV conduction may be increased (conduction time is decreased), ie, paradoxical tachycardia. (**Ref. 1,** pp. 198, 199; **Ref. 3,** p. 425; **Ref. 4,** pp. 854, 855; **Ref. 12,** p. 215)

173. A. In conduction defect arrhythmias, the mechanism of action of class I agents is the conversion of one-way block (retrograde conduction) to two-way block. Digitalis promotes delayed after-depolarization-type of abnormal generation of impulses diagrammed in panel C of Figure 4. Calcium channel blockers alter the slow calcium channel (phase 2). (**Ref. 1,** pp. 194, 195; **Ref. 2,** pp. 282, 283; **Ref. 3,** p. 423; **Ref. 4,** p. 845; **Ref. 12,** pp. 211–212)

174. A. Early after-depolarization is associated with hypoxia, while delayed after-depolarization (panel C) is associated with low potassium, cardiac glycosides, or catecholamines. (**Ref. 2,** p. 280; **Ref. 4,** p.844)

175. D. An increase in dV/dt in phase 4 would lend to aberrant impulses in latent pacemaker tissue, non-pacemaker tissue and also cause spontaneously depolarizing tissue to accelerate. (**Ref. 1,** p.196; **Ref. 3,** pp. 423, 424; **Ref. 4,** p. 847; **Ref. 12,** p. 211)

176. C. The management of chronic congestive heart failure involves both pharmacologic and nonpharmacologic approaches. The pharmacodynamic action of cardiac glycosides, to increase the force of myocardial contraction, is well recognized and has been relied on for treatment of congestive heart failure. (**Ref. 3,** p. 409; **Ref. 6,** p. 732; **Ref. 8,** pp. 815, 830; **Ref. 12,** p. 197)

177. E. The qualitative actions of all digitalis compounds are approximately equal and all have approximately the same therapeutic index. (**Ref. 2,** pp. 261, 262; **Ref. 3,** p. 413; **Ref. 4,** p. 832)

178. C. Because digoxin is not readily metabolized, but is excreted rapidly, and unchanged in the urine, digoxin has a half-life that is dependent in large measure on the adequacy of renal function. Digitoxin is metabolized by the liver, has a long half-life, is readily absorbed, and is extensively protein bound. (**Ref. 1,** pp. 178, 179; **Ref. 2,** p. 258; **Ref. 3,** pp. 414, 415; **Ref. 4,** pp. 828, 829; **Ref. 12,** p. 192)

179. **B.** Digitalis decreases the ventricular rate by prolonging the refractory period of the AV conduction tissue through both direct and vagal effects. (**Ref. 1,** p. 181; **Ref. 2,** p. 261; **Ref. 3,** p. 412; **Ref. 4,** p. 826; **Ref. 12,** p. 194)

180. **D.** Plasma triglyceride concentration is reduced within 5 days of the onset of clofibrate therapy by lowering the levels of very low-density lipoproteins (VLDL). Since a large fall in VLDL may be accompanied by a rise in low-density lipoproteins (LDL), the net effect on cholesterol may be slight. (**Ref. 1,** p. 484; **Ref. 2,** p. 208; **Ref. 3,** p. 489; **Ref. 4,** pp. 874, 886; **Ref. 12,** p. 530)

181. **C.** Cholestyramine is the chloride salt of a quaternary ammonium anion-exchange resin that binds bile acids in the intestine, exchanging them for the chloride ion. This eventually leads to a reduction in LDL due to increased LDL catabolism. (**Ref. 1,** pp. 485, 486; **Ref. 2,** pp. 203, 204; **Ref. 3,** p. 482; **Ref. 4,** p. 840; **Ref. 12,** pp. 530–531)

182. **D.** Atrial fibrillation of recent origin is an indication rather than a contraindication for the use of quinidine. (**Ref. 1,** p. 199; **Ref. 3,** p. 425; **Ref. 4,** pp. 854–856; **Ref. 12,** p. 215)

183. **D.** Cinchonism is caused by cinchona and salicylate. Hypotension, which is the result of peripheral vasodilation, is a consistent effect of quinidine overdosage, especially if the drug is given intravenously. A portion of the hypotensive effect is due to α-receptor blockade. (**Ref. 1,** p. 198; **Ref. 2,** p. 287; **Ref. 3,** p. 425; **Ref. 4,** pp. 855–856; **Ref. 12,** p. 215)

184. **C.** Hydralazine, a direct-acting vascular smooth-muscle relaxant, has not been reported to produce AV block. It has side effects associated with an overextension of its pharmacologic effect and associated with immunologic reactions. Hydralazine is mainly used in combination therapy for severe hypertension. (**Ref. 1,** p. 153; **Ref. 2,** p. 233; **Ref. 3,** p. 176; **Ref. 4,** p. 800; **Ref. 12,** p. 161)

185. **A.** The indirect (vagal) and direct effects of digitalis on AV nodal conduction are synergistic and lead to dose-related depression of AV conduction. (**Ref. 1,** p. 181; **Ref. 4,** pp. 820–821; **Ref. 12,** pp. 193–194)

186. C. Digitalis, by improving cardiac and circulatory function, decreases existing high sympathetic activity, which is a compensatory reflex in congestive failure. (**Ref. 1,** p. 183; **Ref. 3,** p. 412; **Ref. 4,** p. 826; **Ref. 12,** pp. 197–198)

187. B. The angiotensin-converting enzyme inhibitors are useful in treating hypertension with minimal side effects. Hydralazine and minoxidil are direct vasodilators, used for severe hypertension. Propranolol is a β-blocker and prazosin is a selective α_1-antagonist. (**Ref. 1,** pp. 142, 156; **Ref. 2,** p. 230; **Ref. 3,** p. 178; **Ref. 4,** pp. 806–807; **Ref. 12,** p. 163)

188. D. Cardiac glycosides increase automaticity (phase 4) and shorten refractory period (action potential duration/phase 2 and 3). (**Ref. 4,** p. 819)

189. D. Inhibition of Na^+, K^+-ATPase occurs, but it is the exchange of calcium ion that makes contractile calcium available. ATP does not accumulate. All cardiac glycosides act by the same mechanism. (**Ref. 1,** p. 179; **Ref. 2,** p. 259; **Ref. 3,** p. 412, 413; **Ref. 4,** p. 817; **Ref. 12,** p. 192)

190. D. Generation-type arrhythmias can be inhibited by increasing threshold (less negative), increasing resting membrane potential (more negative), and decreasing automaticity (dV/dt phase 4). Choices C and E relate to termination of conduction-type arrhythmias. (**Ref. 1,** p. 194; **Ref. 3,** p. 422; **Ref. 4,** p. 840; **Ref. 12,** p. 210)

191. C. The cardiac arrhythmia suppression test (CAST) demonstrated that class I agents, which are potent sodium channel blockers, should not be used to routinely suppress all arrhythmias. The agents are reserved for life-threatening ventricular arrhythmias. (**Ref. 1,** p. 205; **Ref. 2,** p. 298; **Ref. 3,** p. 431; **Ref. 4,** p.863; **Ref. 12,** pp. 221, 226)

192. C. Intravenous heparin is immediately effective while oral coumadin interferes with clotting factor synthesis. Heparin does not cross into the placenta or into breast milk. However, it should be administered to pregnant women only if a clear need can be demonstrated. (**Ref. 1,** pp. 467, 468; **Ref. 2,** pp. 315–317; **Ref. 3,** pp. 452–455; **Ref. 4,** pp. 1314, 1317; **Ref. 12,** p. 510)

193. **A.** Lovastatin is an inhibitor of the enzyme that synthesizes cholesterol. Cholestyramine binds bile acids and the synthesis of LDL is not influenced by probucol. VLDL secretion is inhibited by nicotinic acid. Lipoprotein lipase is stimulated by clofibrate. (**Ref. 1,** pp. 483–487; **Ref. 4,** pp. 883, 886, 889, 893; **Ref. 12,** pp. 531–532)

194. **A.** Enalapril is an angiotensin converting enzyme (ACE) inhibitor. Methyldopa is converted to α-methylnorepinephrine, which is the α_2-agonist that acts centrally. The inhibition of AChE would be accomplished with neostigmine. (**Ref. 1,** pp. 151, 156; **Ref. 4,** p. 785; **Ref. 12,** p. 164)

195. **C.** Organic nitrates and nitrites cause cGMP formation, leading to nitric oxide formation and dephosphorylation of myosin. (**Ref. 1,** p. 165; **Ref. 4,** p. 768; **Ref. 12,** p. 173)

196. **C.** Quinidine usually produces thrombocytopenia, whereas procainamide has a toxic effect of causing SLE-like syndrome. (**Ref. 1,** pp. 198, 201; **Ref. 4,** pp. 856–857; **Ref. 12,** pp. 215–216)

197. **B.** The most effective agent would be lidocaine to control the accelerated ventricular rate. While hypokalemia might be expected due to the use of thiazides, the patient is ingesting food that contains large amounts of potassium ion. (**Ref. 2,** p. 293; **Ref. 4,** pp. 834, 835; **Ref. 12,** p. 221)

198. **D.** The management of digitalis intoxication includes or may include all of the choices; however, it is often forgotten that administration of the offending agent should cease. (**Ref. 1,** p. 184; **Ref. 2,** p. 262; **Ref. 3,** p. 418; **Ref. 4,** pp. 834–835; **Ref. 12,** p. 198)

199. **E.** In a patient who has been ingesting potassium-containing food, the levels of potassium should be determined before administration of potassium ion. Serum levels of potassium on the order of 4 mEq/L lead to complete AV block and potassium is contraindicated. (**Ref. 2,** p. 263; **Ref. 3,** p. 418; **Ref. 4,** p. 835)

200. **A.** This patient most likely has congestive heart failure, and administration of cardiac glycosides will increase vagal tone, thus slowing the heart rate as well as improving cardiovascular dynam-

ics. This results in the removal of accumulated edema fluid and in improved breathing. (**Ref. 1**, p. 185; **Ref. 2**, p. 261; **Ref. 4**, pp. 830–831; **Ref. 12**, p. 199)

201. D. This patient is not in severe enough distress to warrant intravenous or rapid administration of cardiac glycosides. It is safer to allow adjustments to occur at a slower rate. Unless other factors warrant a change, digoxin would be preferred. (**Ref. 1**, p. 183; **Ref. 2**, p. 262; **Ref. 3**, p. 414; **Ref. 4**, p. 829; **Ref. 12**, pp. 198–199)

202. B. All of the items listed could be an indication of an effect of digitalis, especially toxicity, but the indirect effect of digitalis, which is to increase vagal tone and decrease heart rate, would be noticed first. (**Ref. 1**, p. 185; **Ref. 2**, pp. 261, 262; **Ref. 4**, p. 823, 832; **Ref. 12**, p. 199)

203. E. Withdrawal of cardiac sympathetic tone by administration of the β-blocker propranolol accentuates vagal influences on the heart to increase the degree of AV block. (**Ref. 2**, p. 302; **Ref. 4**, p. 866)

204. A. Phenytoin is used to manage both supraventricular and ventricular ectopic rhythms when digitalis is the causative agent. However, lidocaine is usually preferred. (**Ref. 1**, p. 204; **Ref. 2**, p. 295; **Ref. 4**, p. 854; **Ref. 12**, p. 221)

205. C. In contrast to the minor benefits obtained with digitalis in the so-called high-output failures that occur with AV fistula, thyrotoxicosis, and other conditions, the best results with digitalis cardiac glycosides are obtained in heart failure associated with low cardiac output. (**Ref. 1**, p. 185; **Ref. 2**, p. 261; **Ref. 4**, pp. 830–831; **Ref. 12**, p. 199)

206. D. Adenosine is not conventionally classified as an antiarrhythmic. It has a half-life of 10 seconds and is effective in termination, but not prophylactic treatment, of supraventricular arrhythmias. (**Ref. 1**, p. 207; **Ref. 2**, p. 310; **Ref. 12**, p. 224)

207. C. In contrast to digoxin, which is essentially excreted unchanged in the urine, digitoxin undergoes significant hepatic degradation and enterohepatic recirculation, with approximately 25% of the metabolic end-products appearing in the feces. The serum half-life of digoxin in humans is 1.5 days, whereas the serum half-life of digitoxin is 5 to 7 days. (**Ref. 1,** pp. 178, 179; **Ref. 2,** p. 258; **Ref. 3,** p. 415; **Ref. 4,** pp. 827, 828; **Ref. 12,** p. 192)

208. B. The anion-exchange resin cholestyramine may interfere via binding with the absorption of fat-soluble vitamins, such as K, and numerous drugs, including the cardiac glycosides. (**Ref. 1,** p. 486; **Ref. 2,** p. 204; **Ref. 3,** p. 418; **Ref. 4,** p.851; **Ref. 12,** p. 531)

209. D. Quinidine, through its vagolytic effects, can increase the conductivity of the AV node. (**Ref. 1,** p. 198; **Ref. 3,** p. 425; **Ref. 4,** p. 851; **Ref. 12,** pp. 214–215)

210. A. Amrinone, a bipyridine derivative, increases the force of myocardial contraction and is useful in selected cases of congestive heart failure. It appears that these compounds are specific inhibitors of phosphodiesterase isoform III. (**Ref. 1,** p. 182; **Ref. 2,** p. 263; **Ref. 4,** p. 836; **Ref. 12,** p. 196)

211. B. Amiodarone has been used for a wide spectrum of atrial and ventricular arrhythmias. However, it may produce hepatitis, pulmonary toxicity, and worsening of arrhythmias. It also causes corneal deposits and a bluish color of the skin. (**Ref. 2,** p. 305; **Ref. 4,** pp. 867–868; **Ref. 12,** p. 218)

212. D. Labetalol inhibits α_1-, β_1-, and β_2-adrenergic receptors. (**Ref. 1,** p. 151; **Ref. 2,** p. 142; **Ref. 4,** p. 236; **Ref. 12,** pp. 158–159)

213. C. Tocainide is a class I_B antiarrhythmic agent that causes nausea, vomiting, and neurologic side effects, including tremor and headache. Adverse effects with bretylium include hypotension, gastrointestinal upset, and parotid pain. (**Ref. 1,** p. 204; **Ref. 2,** p. 296; **Ref. 3,** p. 431; **Ref. 4,** pp. 861, 868; **Ref. 12,** p. 221)

214. A. α_1-Acid glycoprotein in the plasma, which binds lidocaine, increases after myocardial infarction. This results in increased levels of lidocaine, but the free active levels do not increase proportionately. (**Ref. 3,** p. 430; **Ref. 4,** p. 851; **Ref. 12,** p. 221)

215. A. When used as a local anesthetic, lidocaine often contains a vasoconstrictor. Preparations for control of arrhythmias by intravenous injection should never contain adrenergic amines. (**Ref. 2,** p. 367; **Ref. 3,** p. 430; **Ref. 4,** p. 860)

216. **A.** Lidocaine is absorbed from the intestinal tract when administered orally; however, most of the lidocaine is metabolized on the first pass through the liver. (**Ref. 1,** p. 204; **Ref. 2,** p. 292; **Ref. 3,** p. 430; **Ref. 4,** pp. 852, 859; **Ref. 12,** p. 220)

217. **C.** If bleeding becomes severe, the use of 1 mg of positively charged protamine will antagonize 100 units of heparin. Mild effects are managed by discontinuing heparin administration. (**Ref. 6,** p. 1344; **Ref. 8,** p. 1317; **Ref. 9,** p. 374; **Ref. 12,** p. 511)

218. **B.** Quinidine prolongs the P wave, the QRS complex, and the T wave in the usual dose and to a greater extent in larger doses. Digoxin does not widen the QRS complex, it shortens the Q-T interval, and flattens or inverts the T wave; with full doses, the P-R interval is lengthened. Lidocaine has negligible effects on the electrocardiogram. Heparin and dicumarol are anticoagulants. (**Ref. 1,** pp. 180, 198; **Ref. 3,** p. 426; **Ref. 4,** pp. 824, 851, 859; **Ref. 12,** pp. 214–215)

219. **A.** The digitalis glycosides reduce end-diastolic volume and increase the force and speed of cardiac contraction. In congestive failure, these two actions are responsible for increased cardiac output. Circulation is improved, venous pressure is reduced, tissue hypoxia is eliminated, edematous fluid is absorbed, and diuresis occurs. (**Ref. 1,** p. 177; **Ref. 2,** p. 259; **Ref. 3,** p. 410; **Ref. 4,** p. 825)

220. **B.** Quinidine toxicity involves paradoxical tachycardia, sudden cardiac death, and various arrhythmias. Many of the toxic effects of quinidine are related to sodium channel blockade or antimuscarinic effects. It also suppresses cardiac force development and must be used with great caution in congestive heart failure. (**Ref. 2,** p. 287; **Ref. 4,** p. 855; **Ref. 5,** p. 626)

221. **A.** All three agents (verapamil, nifedipine, diltiazem) increase blood flow and decrease vascular resistance. Nifedipine has the greatest vasodilator action. Verapamil has the greatest effect on AV conduction. Calcium channel blockers are used for supraven-

tricular arrhythmias. (**Ref. 1**, p. 171; **Ref. 2**, p. 253; **Ref. 3**, p. 445; **Ref. 4**, p. 777; **Ref. 12**, p. 179)

222. **E.** A major side effect of calcium channel blockers is due to vasodilation, which can cause all the effects listed except diarrhea. They may cause constipation. (**Ref. 1**, p. 170; **Ref. 2**, p. 253; **Ref. 3**, p. 445; **Ref. 4**, pp. 778–779, 870; **Ref. 12**, p. 181)

223. **D.** Because minoxidil has little effect on the capacitance vessels, its arterial vasodilation results in reflex sympathetic activation and a threefold increase in cardiac output. An interesting side effect has been increased hair growth. It is combined with a diuretic because it causes sodium and fluid retention. (**Ref. 1**, p. 153; **Ref. 2**, p. 234, 235; **Ref. 4**, pp. 801–802; **Ref. 12**, p. 161)

224. **A.** β-Adrenergic antagonists, calcium channel blockers, and organic nitrates, not nitrites, are considered primary agents for acute management of angina pectoris. An inhibitor of platelet aggregation, aspirin has been shown to reduce the frequency and severity of anginal attacks. (**Ref. 1**, pp. 171–173; **Ref. 4**, p. 764; **Ref. 5**, pp. 613, 622; **Ref. 12**, p. 172)

225. **E.** All of the routes are employed, including oral. However, oral administration is ineffective due to high capacitance organic reductase in the liver. (**Ref. 1**, p.164; **Ref. 2**, p. 268; **Ref. 4**, pp. 769–779; **Ref. 12**, p. 173)

226. **D.** The use of vasodilators usually results in the development of tolerance but their use to acutely increase cardiac output via reduction of the load on the heart is an important aspect of their action. (**Ref. 1**, p. 185; **Ref. 2**, p. 264; **Ref. 4**, pp. 772, 830; **Ref. 12**, pp. 199–200)

227. **E.** In most patients, the QRS complex does not change. It is only in WPW that an increase occurs. Digitalis is contraindicated in WPW. All of the other effects do occur, as well as arrhythmia. (**Ref. 1**, p. 184; **Ref. 4**, p. 824; **Ref. 12**, p. 198)

228. **B.** Cardiac glycosides possess sugar molecules at position 3, which influence solubility, but the basic activity resides in the genin or aglycon. An unsaturated lactone group is necessary at position 17. Naturally occurring cardiac glycosides have hydroxyl at position 14 but neither this hydroxyl nor the sugar are necessary

for biologic activity. (**Ref. 1,** pp. 177, 178; **Ref. 2,** p. 258; **Ref. 3,** p. 413; **Ref. 4,** pp. 814–815; **Ref. 12,** p. 191)

229. **D.** Lidocaine is the drug of first choice for acute management; however, chronic therapy requires an orally-effective agent. Most of the agents available are toxic and may promote arrhythmias. This drug therapy is complicated by the fact that it is not often possible to clearly identify the type of arrhythmia. Sometimes a change in stress level or a dietary change (elimination of caffeine) may eliminate the arrhythmia. Some symptomless or non–life-threatening arrhythmias do not need drug treatment at all. (**Ref. 1,** p. 209; **Ref. 2,** p. 275; **Ref. 12,** p. 225)

230. **C.** Quinidine has strong anticholinergic activity. It stimulates uterine smooth muscle to contract and it also has antipyretic and antimalarial activity. Quinidine is the *d*- isomer of quinine. (**Ref. 1,** p. 198; **Ref. 2,** p. 284; **Ref. 12,** pp. 214–215)

231. **A.** Amiodarone is an antiarrhythmic agent that possesses multiple activities. It blocks sodium channels and it has some β-receptor blocking action. The unique feature of class III antiarrhythmic agents is prolongation of the duration of the action potential. (**Ref. 1,** p. 205; **Ref. 2,** p. 284; **Ref. 4,** pp. 866, 867; **Ref. 12,** p. 219)

232. **D.** Verapamil or propranolol would be preferable agents; however, propranolol may cause exercise intolerance. (**Ref. 1,** p. 207; **Ref. 2,** p. 308; **Ref. 4,** p. 869; **Ref. 12,** p. 224)

233. **E.** Lidocaine blocks both the activated and inactivated sodium channels, in contrast to quinidine, which blocks only the activated channels. This local anesthetic also appears to have most of its effect on damaged tissue rather than "normal" myocardium. A result of quinidine action is a shorter systole and thus a longer diastole, percentage-wise. (**Ref. 1,** p. 203; **Ref. 2,** p. 292; **Ref. 4,** pp. 858, 859; **Ref. 12,** p. 220)

234. **B.** Clonidine belongs to a newer group of antihypertensive agents which are α_2-agonists. These compounds act centrally to inhibit sympathetic outflow. Methyldopa also acts through this central mechanism. It is converted to α-methylnorepinephrine which is a potent α_2-agonist. (**Ref. 1,** p. 144; **Ref. 2,** p. 246; **Ref. 4,** p. 791; **Ref. 12,** p. 153)

235. A. Metyrosine inhibits the conversion of tyrosine to DOPA by acting on tyrosine hydroxylase. It has limited usefulness in the management of pheochromocytoma.(**Ref. 1,** p. 128; **Ref. 2,** p. 244; **Ref. 4,** p. 796; **Ref. 12,** pp. 136–137)

236. D. Ganglionic-blocking agents have such widespread side effects that their use is restricted to malignant hypertension. However, trimetaphan can be infused in a hypertensive crisis or used for controlled hypotension during surgery. Its effect only lasts approximately 15 minutes. (**Ref. 1,** p. 146; **Ref. 2,** p. 244; **Ref. 4,** p. 793; **Ref. 12,** p. 154)

237. E. Guanethidine has multiple effects on sympathetic nerve endings. It decreases adrenergic amine stores in the nerve ending after initially releasing norepinephrine. Its antihypertensive action in severe hypertension most likely results from inhibition of the release of adrenergic amines from the nerve ending in a manner similar but not identical to that of bretylium. However, it must first enter the nerve ending and uptake$_1$ inhibitors will block the action of guanethidine by preventing its access to the nerve. (**Ref. 1,** p. 147; **Ref. 2,** pp. 240, 241; **Ref. 4,** p. 794; **Ref. 12,** p. 155)

238. D. Withdrawal of β-adrenergic blocking agents must always be done cautiously. Up-regulation of receptors occurs and time must be given for a readjustment to occur. These agents are not vasodilators, are not useful in vasospastic angina (may worsen it) and most β-blockers are both effective and used in combination with organic nitrates. (**Ref. 1,** p. 172; **Ref. 2,** pp. 272, 273; **Ref. 4,** p. 780; **Ref. 12,** p. 182)

239. E. Abnormal rhythms can occur due to abnormal conduction, abnormal generation (ectopic pacemakers, spontaneous depolarization). Cardiac glycosides, β-adrenergic blocking agents, or calcium channel blockers will protect the ventricle from aberrant impulses. Catecholamines may eliminate unidirectional conduction, but would increase generation arrhythmias. (**Ref. 1,** pp. 194, 195; **Ref. 4,** pp. 843–846)

240. C. While angiotensin converting enzyme inhibitors are relatively safe agents, they cause a decrease in angiotensin, which is necessary for renal perfusion in bilateral renal artery stenosis; they are thus contraindicated in this condition. (**Ref. 1,** p. 157; **Ref. 2,** p. 193; **Ref. 4,** pp. 759, 761; **Ref. 12,** p. 165)

241. C. The second-generation activators of plasminogen are more effective when the binding of fibrin has occurred. This provides a fibrin-selective activation of plasminogen. This activation of plasminogen is not absolute. (**Ref. 1,** p. 471; **Ref. 2,** p. 322; **Ref. 4,** pp. 1322–1324; **Ref. 12,** p. 515)

242. A. Bleeding is the major complication of using heparin. It does not cross the placenta, which is in contrast to oral anticoagulants. Mild elevation of hepatic transaminases occurs, allergic reactions occur rarely, and aldosterone-synthesis inhibition occurs occasionally. (**Ref. 2,** p. 316; **Ref. 4,** p. 1316; **Ref. 12,** p. 509)

243. A. All of the interactions occur except the cimetidine choice. Cimetidine does not stimulate, it inhibits, the hepatic metabolism of quinidine. Elevated levels of quinidine are observed. (**Ref. 2,** p. 287)

244. B. Tocainide and mexiletine are orally effective congeners of lidocaine that are useful for ventricular arrhythmias. They are I_B agents. Procainamide results when the ester procaine is changed to an amide. Disopyramide has antimuscarinic effects similar to those of atropine. Amiodarone is a class III antiarrhythmic. Esmolol is a short acting β-adrenergic blocking agent. (**Ref. 1,** pp. 202, 204; **Ref. 2,** p. 296; **Ref. 4,** pp. 851, 861; **Ref. 12,** p. 221)

245. E. The VLDL-lowering action of niacin that occurs at very high doses is not related to its action as a vitamin. This large concentration produces an intense cutaneous flush and this leads to decreased patient acceptance. (**Ref. 1,** pp. 481, 483; **Ref. 2,** pp. 204, 205; **Ref. 4,** p. 893; **Ref. 12,** p. 529)

246. C. Thrombocytopenia is an adverse reaction associated with quinidine. A large number of patients receiving procainamide will have antinuclear antibodies and a portion of that group will develop an SLE-like syndrome. (**Ref. 1,** pp. 200, 201; **Ref. 2,** p. 288; **Ref. 4,** p. 856; **Ref. 12,** p. 216)

247. D. Cardiac glycosides have a structure similar to that of the estrogen molecule. It is postulated that the unusual side effect of gynecomastia in males is related to estrogenic activity. (**Ref. 1,** p. 184; **Ref. 2,** p. 262; **Ref. 4,** p. 834; **Ref. 12,** p. 195)

248. **A.** Urokinase directly activates plasminogen, in contrast to streptokinase, which must bind to proactivator plasminogen. With streptokinase bound to the proactivator, inactive plasminogen is converted to active plasminogen. Tissue-plasminogen activator activates plasminogen bound to fibrin. Streptokinase comes from streptococci. Urokinase is obtained from human kidney cell culture, and is better tolerated. (**Ref. 1,** p. 471; **Ref. 2,** pp. 321, 322; **Ref. 4,** pp. 1323, 1324; **Ref. 12,** p. 515)

249. **B.** Heparin releases lipoprotein lipase from endothelial cells and clears lipids from the serum. This anticoagulant is antagonized by protamine. It acts both in vitro and in vivo. (**Ref. 1,** p. 467; **Ref. 2,** p. 315; **Ref. 4,** p. 1315; **Ref. 12,** p. 509)

250. **D.** Saralasin is an angiotensin peptide analog that competitively inhibits angiotensin receptors. It has a short half-life (3 minutes). Given intravenously, it has been proposed as a diagnostic aid to diagnose angiotensin-dependent hypertension. (**Ref. 1,** p. 156; **Ref. 2,** p. 194; **Ref. 12,** p. 163)

251. **C.** Oral anticoagulants inhibit vitamin K. Vitamin K catalyzes the conversion of precursors to vitamin K-dependent clotting factors. Administration of vitamin K_1 (phytonadione) will restore clotting in 24 hours. Immediate reversal is obtained by administration of plasma containing vitamin K-dependent factors. (**Ref. 1,** p. 473; **Ref. 2,** p. 317; **Ref. 4,** pp. 1317, 1320; **Ref. 12,** pp. 517–518)

252. **E.** The aldosterone-antagonist spironolactone is structurally related to aldosterone, enabling it to act as a competitive inhibitor of aldosterone. It is only effective when mineralocorticoids are present. (**Ref. 1,** pp. 222, 223; **Ref. 2,** pp. 224, 225; **Ref. 4,** pp. 725, 726; **Ref. 12,** pp. 241–242)

253. **E.** Spironolactone is used in patients who have low serum potassium and cannot tolerate potassium supplementation or are unable to tolerate oral potassium. (**Ref. 1,** pp. 222, 223; **Ref. 2,** pp. 224, 225; **Ref. 4,** pp. 725, 726; **Ref. 12,** pp. 241–242)

5

Drugs Affecting Metabolic and Endocrine Functions

DIRECTIONS (Questions 253–273): Each of the questions or incomplete statements below is followed by five suggested answers or completions. Select the **one** that is best in each case.

253. Androgens will do all of the following EXCEPT
  A. stimulate erythropoietin production
  B. provide specific androgenic effects without anabolic action
  C. provide palliative relief of advanced inoperable cancer of the breast in postmenopausal patients
  D. increase muscle mass and body weight in hypogonadism
  E. treat mild anemia

254. All of the following statements concerning progesterone are true EXCEPT
  A. it causes a secretory endometrium following estrogen priming
  B. it binds to a specific cytosolic receptor
  C. administration leads to a decrease in body temperature
  D. it is too rapidly absorbed from oily solutions to be of optimal benefit
  E. it is secreted mainly in the second half of the menstrual cycle

255. All of the following are adverse effects of oral contraceptives EXCEPT
   A. an increased incidence of cardiovascular disease with combined products
   B. breast engorgement and discomfort
   C. hypertension
   D. CNS stimulation and increased endurance
   E. changes in the plasma concentrations of lipids

256. All of the following statements regarding sulfonylurea antidiabetic drugs are true EXCEPT
   A. drug sensitivity occurs in 1% to 5% of patients and cross-sensitivity among these drugs is common
   B. patients who drink alcoholic beverages while taking these drugs may experience a disulfiram-like reaction
   C. hypoglycemic reactions are more common among mild diabetics and may recur several days later even though the drug has been discontinued
   D. serious hematopoietic and hepatic effects occur only rarely
   E. when they are administered orally, the duration of action of all of these drugs is similar

257. Regarding isophane (NPH) insulin, all of the following statements are true EXCEPT
   A. it is considered an intermediate-acting insulin
   B. it has a rapid intense action that starts about 2 hours following administration and reaches its peak of activity in 8–10 hours
   C. after 10 hours it slowly has less effect, so that at 24 hours it has very little if any effect
   D. isophane and regular insulin can be premixed in syringes and stored for 30 days in the refrigerator
   E. it is used in treating all diabetic states except for the initial management of diabetic ketoacidosis or diabetic emergencies

258. The mineralocorticoid activity of some of the anti-inflammatory steroids would be most likely to induce
   A. peptic ulcer
   B. hypokalemic alkalosis
   C. psychosis
   D. buffalo hump
   E. abdominal striae

259. Mestranol exerts its contraceptive action primarily by
   A. inhibiting follicle-stimulating hormone (FSH) secretion
   B. inhibiting luteinizing hormone (LH) secretion
   C. stimulating FSH secretion
   D. stimulating LH secretion
   E. inhibiting transportation of spermatozoa to the ovum

260. Chronic treatment with large doses of prednisolone may result in all of the following EXCEPT
   A. reduction of endogenous secretion of adrenocorticotropic hormone (ACTH)
   B. increased susceptibility to infections
   C. hyperglycemia and glycosuria
   D. fluid and electrolyte disturbances
   E. increased bone density

261. Corticosteroids are usually indicated in all of the following conditions EXCEPT
   A. herpes simplex of the eye
   B. status asthmaticus
   C. nephrotic syndrome
   D. collagen diseases
   E. chronic adrenal insufficiency

262. Regarding drugs affecting fertility, all of the following statements are true EXCEPT
   A. clomiphene promotes fertility in anovulatory women
   B. in combination oral contraceptives, the progestin is added primarily to stimulate the secretion of LH
   C. ethinyl estradiol possesses high oral estrogenic potency
   D. combination oral contraceptives containing high doses of estrogens can alter glucose tolerance
   E. estrogen promotes closure of the epiphyses of long bones

263. The physiologic and pharmacologic actions of estrogens include all of the following EXCEPT
    A. they cause growth and development of the vagina, uterus, and fallopian tubes
    B. they promote ductile growth of the breasts
    C. the increase of estrogenic activity at the end of the menstrual cycle induces menstruation
    D. estrogens can promote salt and water retention
    E. regional pigmentation of the areola and nipples is induced by estrogens

264. All of the following facts about prolactin are true EXCEPT
    A. prolactin does not currently have a defined therapeutic use
    B. bromocriptine will inhibit prolactin secretion
    C. hyperprolactinemia may result in amenorrhea or galactorrhea
    D. there are specific receptors for prolactin in numerous tissues other than the mammary gland
    E. prolactin is an antagonist of growth hormone

265. Corticotropin-releasing hormone (CRH)
    A. releases thyroxine from the thyroid gland
    B. releases ACTH from the pituitary
    C. releases glucocorticoids from the adrenal gland
    D. is a potentiator of hydrocortisone at tissue sites
    E. releases somatostatin

266. Thyroid hormones
    A. inhibit growth
    B. decrease metabolism
    C. are not considered calorigenic
    D. inhibit thyroid-stimulating hormone (TSH) release
    E. tend to decrease cardiac output

267. Hypothyroidism is preferentially treated with
    A. synthetic T_4
    B. synthetic T_3
    C. desiccated thyroid (T_3 and T_4)
    D. subcutaneous T_4
    E. intravenous T_3

268. Propylthiouracil
   A. accumulates in the thyroid gland
   B. stimulates thyroid hormone formation
   C. causes the thyroid gland to shrink
   D. inhibits active iodine transport
   E. causes iodine to accumulate in thyroglobulin

269. All of the following statements about oral contraceptives are true EXCEPT
   A. the risk factors should be evaluated for all patients
   B. patients above 30 years of age tend to have fewer risk factors
   C. oral contraceptives frequently cause nausea, dizziness, breast discomfort, and weight gain
   D. "pill" users have an increased risk of coronary thrombosis
   E. hypertension may occur in a segment of the population using oral contraceptives

270. Except for specific therapy, contraindications for the use of estrogens includes all of the following EXCEPT
   A. endometrial cancer
   B. breast cancer
   C. liver disease
   D. thromboembolic disorder
   E. kidney disease

271. Corticosteroids
   A. possess either mineralocorticoid or glucocorticoid activity
   B. may cause severe inflammatory responses
   C. stimulate protein synthesis
   D. cause fluid retention and edema
   E. may produce hypoglycemia

272. The primary factor that regulates the secretory activity of the parathyroid gland under physiologic conditions is the
   A. concentration of ionized calcium in the circulation
   B. blood concentration of extracellular phosphate ion
   C. concentration of circulating calcitonin in the region of the gland
   D. vitamin D concentration in parathyroid cells
   E. blood concentration of a tropic hormone secreted by the anterior pituitary

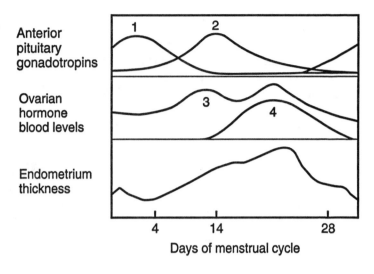

Figure 7

273. Referring to Figure 7, which of the following statements is INCORRECT

   A. Ovulation occurs at about day 14 of the menstrual cycle
   B. The pituitary gonadotropic hormone peaking at site 2 is prolactin, which precipitates menses
   C. The ovarian hormone that peaks at site 3 is estrogen
   D. The anterior pituitary gonadotropin that peaks at site 1 is follicle-stimulating hormone (FSH) which, in addition to stimulating follicle growth and enlargement of the ovum, increases proliferation of theca cells, which produce estrogen.
   E. The ovarian hormone peaking at site 4 is progesterone, which is of primary importance in the development of a secretory endometrium

---

DIRECTIONS (Questions 274–296): Each group of questions below consists of five lettered headings followed by a list of numbered phrases or statements. For each numbered phrase or statement, select the **one** lettered heading that is most closely associated with it. Each lettered heading may be selected once, more than once, or not at all.

Questions 274–276:
- **A.** Aldosterone
- **B.** Bromocriptine
- **C.** Carbimazole
- **D.** Tamoxifen
- **E.** Hydrocortisone

274. Used to manage acromegaly

275. Most likely to increase susceptibility to bacterial infection

276. An antiestrogen

Questions 277 and 278:
- **A.** Calcium
- **B.** Calcitonin
- **C.** Sodium etidronate
- **D.** Vitamin D
- **E.** Fluoride

277. A hormone that acts to stimulate absorption of calcium and phosphate from the intestine

278. Orally effective compound for the management of Paget's disease

Questions 279–281:
- **A.** Calcitonin
- **B.** Propranolol
- **C.** Lugol's solution (strong iodide solution)
- **D.** Radioactive iodine
- **E.** Methimazole

279. Its usefulness in treatment of hyperthyroidism is the result of inhibition of thyroid peroxidase and blockade of thyroid peroxidase-catalyzed iodination of thyroglobulin

280. Valuable in controlling symptoms of thyrotoxicosis while awaiting the response to radioiodine and may be useful in treating patients experiencing thyroid storm

281. Large doses paradoxically cause rapid inhibition of thyroid hormone secretion in euthyroid and hyperthyroid individuals—an action that may be responsible for its usefulness in treating Graves' disease

Questions 282–286:
A. Aldosterone
B. Prednisone
C. Dexamethasone
D. Flunisolide
E. Metyrapone

282. Inhibits cytochrome P450 enzymes.

283. Prototype mineralocorticoid

284. A steroid given by inhalation

285. A glucocorticoid used orally that has a long duration of action relative to other agents

286. Reduced in the liver to a compound with approximately the same activity

Questions 287–290:
A. Tolbutamide
B. Glipizide
C. NPH insulin
D. Glucagon
E. Ultralente insulin

287. A second generation sulfonylurea

288. May be used for severe hypoglycemia

289. This compound has a long (24 hours) duration of action and very slow (6 hours) onset of action

290. A compound that is reported to increase cardiovascular mortality when compared to insulin

Questions 291–294:
  A. Androgens
  B. Estrogens
  C. Androgens and estrogens
  D. Neither androgens nor estrogens
  E. Clomiphene

291. Exerts an inhibitory action on cephalic hair growth in females

292. Augments fusion of the epiphyses

293. Synthesized by the ovary

294. Increases libido in normal men

Questions 295 and 296:
  A. Single dose of 1 mg of *l*-triiodothyronine
  B. Single dose of 4 mg of *l*-thyroxine
  C. A single dose of either A or B above
  D. Neither A nor B above
  E. Propranolol

295. Metabolic response occurs in 4 to 6 hours

296. The effect outlasts the presence of detectable elevated amounts of hormone in the blood

---

DIRECTIONS (Questions 297–298): Each of the questions or incomplete statements below is followed by five suggested answers or completions. Select the **one** that is best in each case.

---

297. Estrogenic activity
  A. is exhibited by compounds formed exclusively in the gonads, placenta, and adrenal cortices
  B. is evidenced by compounds with steroidal structure only
  C. is found in the urine of pregnant humans, pregnant mares, and stallions
  D. of the three main human estrogens is highest in estriol
  E. is inhibited by cyclic AMP

298. Administration of therapeutically effective doses of iodide:
   A. stimulates iodination of thyroglobulin
   B. is slow in onset usually taking from 5 to 7 days
   C. destroys the thyroid gland specifically
   D. reduces vascularity of the thyroid gland
   E. is useful for long-term management of hyperthyroidism

DIRECTIONS (Questions 299–300): The group of questions below consists of five lettered headings followed by a list of numbered phrases or statements. For each numbered phrase or statement, select the **one** lettered heading that is most closely associated with it. Each lettered heading may be selected once, more than once, or not at all.

Questions 299 and 300:
   A. Tolbutamide
   B. Chlorpropamide
   C. Acetohexamide
   D. Tolazamide
   E. Phenformin

299. Undergoes rapid biotransformation to active metabolites that extend its duration of action

300. A first-generation sulfonylurea with a biologic half-life of approximately 35 hours

---

DIRECTIONS (Questions 301–306): Each of the questions or incomplete statements below is followed by five suggested answers or completions. Select the **one** that is best in each case.

---

301. All of the following statements regarding insulin/diabetes are true EXCEPT
   A. hypophysectomy ameliorates diabetes mellitus
   B. glucose administered intravenously brings about greater secretion of insulin than when it is given orally
   C. in the human, the normal pancreas produces from 30 to 50 units of insulin daily
   D. polydipsia, polyuria, and polyphagia are among obvious clinical symptoms of diabetes
   E. in healthy individuals the liver and the kidneys are the main sites of biodegradation of insulin

DRUGS AFFECTING BLOOD AND BLOOD-FORMING ORGANS

302. When iron is to be given parenterally
  A. the intramuscular route is the most desirable avenue of administration
  B. the most serious side effects that are likely to be encountered when given intravenously are generalized lymphadenopathy and arthralgias
  C. the preparation most widely used in the United States is iron dextran injection
  D. the intramuscular route affords a highly desirable repository form of iron since > 70% of such a dose may become fixed locally in the muscle for many months
  E. one may be certain that iron so administered will produce a pharmacologic response more rapidly than if it is given orally

303. Most iron in the body is found
  A. in the protein hemoglobin
  B. in the globulin transferrin
  C. in myoglobin
  D. in ferritin, the storage form of iron in tissues
  E. in cytochrome enzymes

304. All of the following statements concerning vitamin B_{12} are true EXCEPT
  A. it is not inherently present in higher plants
  B. man depends on exogenous sources of supply
  C. it is preferentially stored in parenchymal cells of the liver, and the supply of vitamin B_{12} available for tissues is directly related to the size of the hepatic storage pool
  D. intracellular B_{12} is maintained as two active coenzymes, methylcobalamin and deoxyadenosylcobalamin
  E. in humans, the daily nutritional requirement is provided by synthesis in the GI tract

305. Which of the following statements concerning erythropoietin is NOT true?
  A. Erythropoietin is effective in treating anemia of chronic renal failure
  B. The action of erythropoietin is receptor mediated
  C. There is a high incidence of allergic reactions when erythropoietin is administered
  D. There is a constant level of erythropoietin in the plasma
  E. Cancer chemotherapy-induced anemia can be treated with erythropoietin

306. In hematopoiesis
  A. growth factors are very specific for cell type
  B. growth factors have limited action at one part of the proliferation process
  C. growth factors exert delicate control of both hematopoiesis and lymphopoiesis
  D. the process of proliferation of colony-forming units is under exclusive control of IL-2
  E. at steady state the level of blood cells produced is less than 200 million per day

---

DIRECTIONS (Questions 307–312): Each group of questions below consists of five lettered headings followed by a list of numbered phrases or statements. For each numbered phrase or statement, select the **one** lettered heading that is most closely associated with it. Each lettered heading may be selected once, more than once, or not at all.

Questions 307–309:
  A. Vitamin B_{12}
  B. Folic acid
  C. Ferrous sulfate
  D. Heparin
  E. Tissue plasminogen activator (t-PA)

307. A thrombolytic agent

308. A characteristic of this compound is the electronegative charge

309. In a deficiency state, only the megaloblastic anemia, but not the neurologic symptoms, are corrected by this agent

Questions 310–312:
   A. Granulocyte/macrophage colony-stimulating factor (GM-CSF)
   B. Heparin
   C. Aspirin
   D. G-CSF
   E. Streptokinase

310. Administration leads to an increase in circulating neutrophils, monocytes, and eosinophils.

311. Permanent inhibitor of thromboxane A_2 (TXA_2) production

312. Routinely used to inhibit clot formation in tubing and cannulae

---

DIRECTIONS (Questions 313–319): Each of the questions or incomplete statements below is followed by five suggested answers or completions. Select the **one** that is best in each case.

---

313. The mechanism of action of the anticoagulant effect of coumarin derivatives involves
   A. a reduction in levels of factors VII, IX, and X
   B. an action taking place in the bloodstream
   C. no effect on vitamin K
   D. an action that blocks the release of preformed prothrombin by the liver
   E. fibrinolysis

314. Regarding the therapeutic uses of iron
   A. oral ferrous sulfate is the treatment of choice for iron deficiency
   B. ferrous and ferric salts differ very little in their bioavailability
   C. enteric-coated tablets are better absorbed than immediate-release tablets
   D. medicinal iron preparations are relatively nontoxic for children
   E. side effects associated with oral iron therapy include increased sensitivity of the skin to ultraviolet light

VITAMINS

315. Photophobia, lacrimation, stomatitis, cheilosis, and keratitis characterize a deficiency of
A. ascorbic acid
B. vitamin B_2
C. vitamin B_6
D. vitamin D
E. cyanocobalamin

316. Regarding vitamins, all of the following statements are true EXCEPT
A. vitamin deficiency is usually not specific for one vitamin but is a nutritional deficiency in which several vitamins are lacking
B. vitamin supplementation is not generally necessary except for defined special-risk groups, such as in pregnancy and in the elderly
C. fat soluble vitamins include A, C, D, E, and K
D. the term vitamin refers to chemical substances that are necessary in small amounts for growth, metabolism, and development
E. water-soluble vitamins are rapidly metabolized and excreted in the urine

317. All of the following facts about vitamin A are true EXCEPT
A. it improves vision in dim light
B. it is useful in the prophylaxis of certain malignancies
C. different forms of the molecule mediate different functions
D. epithelial cell differentiation is inhibited by vitamin A
E. large tissue reserves are present and deficiency is not noted until deprivation is of long-standing duration

318. Vitamin C
A. megadoses are useful in preventing the common cold
B. prevents kidney stones
C. is necessary for collagen synthesis
D. is low in fresh fruits
E. is another name for folic acid

319. All of the following statements about vitamin D are correct EXCEPT
  A. the major role of vitamin D is to provide a positive influence on calcium ion
  B. vitamin D_3 is formed in the skin
  C. the major source of vitamin D in humans is skin irradiation by sunlight
  D. the principal result of vitamin D deficiency is scurvy
  E. hypervitaminosis D is characterized by hypercalcemia

320. Vitamin A toxicity may cause
  A. teratogenicity
  B. renal stones
  C. impairment of pain, touch, and temperature sensation
  D. flushing and GI disturbances
  E. bleeding

321. Vitamin E is
  A. riboflavin
  B. isotriniton
  C. carotene
  D. biotin
  E. α-tocopherol

322. Vitamin D (cholecalciferol)
  A. is obtained from the diet
  B. is converted to the hormone 7-dehydrocholesterol
  C. is also known as 25-hydroxy D_3, which is devoid of biologic activity
  D. circulates freely in the blood
  E. is eventually converted to 1,25-dihydroxy D_3, the most active form of the vitamin

Drugs Affecting Metabolic and Endocrine Functions

Answers and Discussion

253. **B.** All natural and synthetic androgens have both androgenic and anabolic activity. The ratio of androgenic to anabolic properties differs, depending on the steroid or steroid preparation in question. (**Ref. 1,** p. 578; **Ref. 3,** p. 554; **Ref. 4,** p. 1418; **Ref. 12,** p. 629)

254. **C.** Progesterone causes an increase in body temperature. The mechanism for this is unknown but believed to be associated with an alteration of the temperature-regulating centers in the hypothalamus. This increase in temperature is often used to determine the time of ovulation for the purpose of increasing the likelihood of conception. (**Ref. 1,** p. 565; **Ref. 4,** p. 1399; **Ref. 12,** p. 616)

255. **D.** Oral contraceptives are known to cause depression, fatigue, and lack of initiative. These effects may be lessened by using a product containing a smaller amount of progestin. (**Ref. 1,** pp. 571–573; **Ref. 3,** pp. 551–552; **Ref. 4,** pp. 1406–1408; **Ref. 12,** pp. 622–623)

256. **E.** The duration of action of sulfonylureas is as follows: tolbutamide 6–12 hours, tolazamide 10–14 hours, acetohexamide 12–24 hours, chlorpropamide up to 60 hours, glyburide 10–24 hours, and glipizide 10–24 hours. All sulfonylureas have the

same type of activity and individual agents are chosen based on side effects and patient response. (**Ref. 1**, p. 595; **Ref. 3**, p. 568; **Ref. 4**, pp. 1485–1486; **Ref. 12**, p. 648)

257. **D.** Regular and NPH insulin can be mixed in the same syringe; however, it should be used immediately to prevent binding of the zinc and protamine in the NPH insulin with the regular insulin. (**Ref. 1**, p. 592; **Ref. 4**, p. 1477; **Ref. 10**, p. 2046; **Ref. 12**, p. 643)

258. **B.** Mineralocorticoids favor the retention of sodium and water excretion of potassium, leading to hypokalemic alkalosis and edema. (**Ref. 1**, p. 551; **Ref. 3**, p. 531; **Ref. 4**, p. 1439; **Ref. 12**, p. 602)

259. **A.** The predominant effect of the synthetic estrogen, mestranol, and all estrogens used in oral contraceptives is to inhibit the secretion of FSH by a negative feedback mechanism. (**Ref. 1**, p. 570; **Ref. 3**, pp. 547–48; **Ref. 4**, pp. 1404–1405; **Ref. 10**, p. 2016; **Ref. 12**, p. 608)

260. **E.** Osteoporosis, a frequent serious complication of prolonged corticosteroid therapy, is an indication for withdrawal of therapy. Glucocorticoids inhibit the activity of osteoblasts directly, and through their effects on calcium and parathyroid hormone stimulate the activity of osteoclasts. This results in decreased bone formation and increased bone resorption. (**Ref. 1**, p. 550; **Ref. 3**, p. 532; **Ref. 4**, p. 1452; **Ref. 12**, p. 600)

261. **A.** Corticosteroids are contraindicated in herpes simplex of the eye and in all cases of bacterial, viral, or fungal conjunctivitis because progression of the disease and irreversible clouding of the cornea may occur. (**Ref. 1**, p. 551; **Ref. 4**, p. 1456; **Ref. 10**, p. 1986; **Ref. 12**, pp. 600)

262. **B.** Progestin suppresses ovulation by inhibition of LH through negative feedback on the hypothalamic anterior pituitary axis. (**Ref. 3**, p. 551; **Ref. 4**, p. 1405; **Ref. 10**, p. 2016)

263. **C.** A decline in estrogenic activity at the end of the menstrual cycle actually brings about menstruation. (**Ref. 1**, pp. 559–560; **Ref. 4**, p. 1386; **Ref. 10**, p. 2026; **Ref. 12**, pp. 608–609)

264. E. Prolactin receptors are similar in structure to receptors for growth hormone. Both growth hormone and placental lactogen are agonists at prolactin receptors; however, prolactin is not capable of binding to growth hormone receptors. **(Ref. 4,** p. 1345)

265. B. Corticotropin releasing hormone (CRH) mediates an individual's response to stress through activation of the pituitary-adrenal axis. CRH is used clinically to test for abnormalities in the hypothalamic-pituitary-adrenal axis. **(Ref. 1,** p. 518; **Ref. 3,** p. 521; **Ref. 4,** p. 1356; **Ref. 12,** p. 567)

266. D. With the exception of TSH release, which is inhibited (negative feedback), the calorigenic hormones T_4 and/or T_3, stimulate growth and metabolism. Cardiac output is increased when thyroid levels are elevated. **(Ref. 1,** pp. 530, 533; **Ref. 3,** pp. 574–575; **Ref. 4,** p. 1367; **Ref. 12,** p. 582)

267. A. Thyroid hormones are orally effective and are normally administered by mouth except in myxedema coma, where intravenous T_3 is used. T_4 is the preferred agent. **(Ref. 1,** p. 534; **Ref. 3,** p. 577; **Ref. 4,** pp. 1371–1372; **Ref. 12,** pp. 586–587)

268. A. Antithyroid drugs like propylthiouracil and methimazole accumulate in the gland and inhibit iodination of thyroglobulin. These agents do not block iodine transport. The gland may undergo hypertrophy. **(Ref. 10,** p. 2018; **Ref. 12,** p. 584)

269. B. The use of oral contraceptives is associated with a number of serious adverse effects on the cardiovascular system along with some troublesome effects such as nausea, headache, and some symptoms resembling early pregnancy. Overall, in patients below the age of 30 who do not have risk factors such as hypertension, hyperlipidemia, obesity and diabetes, they are relatively safe. **(Ref. 4,** pp. 1406–1409; **Ref. 10,** p. 2017; **Ref. 12,** pp. 622–623)

270. E. It is recognized that estrogens should not be used in cancer or suspected cancer even though some forms of cancer respond favorably to high doses of estrogen. Thromboembolism or liver disease are also contraindications but there is no evidence they are contraindicated in kidney disease. **(Ref. 1,** p. 564; **Ref. 3,** p. 548; **Ref. 4,** p. 1409; **Ref. 12,** pp. 623–624)

271. D. Corticosteroids have anti-inflammatory activity and metabolic effects resulting in decreased protein synthesis (negative nitrogen balance) and hyperglycemia. All corticosteroids have some degree of glucocorticoid and mineralocorticoid activity. **(Ref. 1,** pp. 545–546; **Ref. 3,** pp. 530–532; **Ref. 4,** pp. 1437–1441; **Ref. 12,** pp. 592, 596)

272. A. Although it is not clear whether the extracellular calcium or the ionized calcium in the parathyroid cells is the actual "trigger" for release of the hormone, the output of parathyroid hormone is apparently regulated by the level of serum calcium acting through a feedback mechanism. **(Ref. 1,** p. 603; **Ref. 3,** p. 584; **Ref. 4,** pp. 1504–1505; **Ref. 12,** pp. 655–656)

273. B. The hormone surging at site 2 is luteinizing hormone. Prolactin is principally responsible for lactation, and its role in the menstrual cycle is unclear. **(Ref. 1,** pp. 523, 560; **Ref. 3,** p. 542; **Ref. 4,** pp. 1344, 1348, 1387; **Ref. 12,** pp. 572, 608–609)

274. B. Tumors of the pituitary that excrete excessive growth hormone can be inhibited by dopaminergic agonists, such as bromocriptine. Its use is associated with a decrease in excessive sweating, a reduction in soft-tissue thickening, an improvement in facial features, and an improvement in glucose tolerance. **(Ref. 1,** p. 524; **Ref. 4,** p. 1346; **Ref. 10,** p. 2433; **Ref. 12,** p. 572)

275. E. Glucocorticoids impair defense mechanisms against infections and increase susceptibility to bacterial and fungal pathogens. This is most common in patients receiving large doses of systemic therapy. **(Ref. 1,** p. 545; **Ref. 4,** p. 1448; **Ref. 10,** pp. 1984–1985; **Ref. 12,** p. 595)

276. D. Tamoxifen is an antiestrogen used in palliative treatment of advanced breast cancer in postmenopausal women. It has also been proven effective as adjuvant treatment in pre- and postmenopausal women with estrogen-receptor or progestin-receptor–positive tumors. **(Ref. 1,** pp. 574, 793; **Ref. 4,** pp. 1256–1257; **Ref. 10,** pp. 689–690; **Ref. 12,** pp. 624, 841)

277. D. Vitamin D is now recognized as a hormone. It increases absorption of calcium and phosphate from the gut, decreases their excretion, and enhances bone resorption. Parathyroid hormone increases intestinal absorption indirectly through calcitriol and directly through an unknown mechanism. (Ref. 1, pp. 603–604; Ref. 4, p. 1510; Ref. 10, p. 2409; Ref. 12, p. 656)

278. **C.** Sodium etidronate has an advantage over calcitonin in that it is inexpensive, orally effective, and less antigenic. Its exact mechanism of action is unknown, but it acts to reduce normal and abnormal bone resorption and to reduce bone formation and turnover. **(Ref. 1,** p. 615; **Ref. 4,** p. 1509; **Ref. 10,** p. 2452; **Ref. 12,** pp. 659–660)

279. **E.** Thioamides such as propylthiouracil and methimazole compete with tyrosine residues of thyroglobulin for active iodine and for inactive thyroid peroxidase. In addition, propylthiouracil, to a greater extent than methimazole, inhibits peripheral deiodination of T_3 and T_4. **(Ref. 1,** p. 535; **Ref. 4,** p. 1374; **Ref. 12,** pp. 587–588)

280. **B.** The increased heart rate, palpitation, anxiety, tension, tremor, and stare associated with hyperthyroidism are rapidly controlled by oral administration of propranolol. **(Ref. 1,** p. 540; **Ref. 4,** p. 1376; **Ref. 10,** p. 1052; **Ref. 12,** p. 589)

281. **C.** Iodide is the first substance known to have been used successfully in the treatment of thyroid disorders, an effect that remains paradoxical, since increased iodide intake would be expected to increase, rather than decrease, thyroid hormone synthesis. **(Ref. 1,** p. 536; **Ref. 4,** p. 1377; **Ref. 10,** p. 1760; **Ref. 12,** p. 589)

282. **E.** Metyrapone is an inhibitor of glucocorticoid synthesis, leading to increased ACTH production. It can be used to test pituitary function and to suppress excess glucocorticoid production in specific situations. **(Ref. 1,** p. 555; **Ref. 4,** p. 1458; **Ref. 10,** p. 1577; **Ref. 12,** p. 604)

283. **A.** Aldosterone is the most potent glucocorticoid synthesized by the adrenal cortex that influences salt and water balance. **(Ref. 1,** p. 552; **Ref. 4,** p. 1431; **Ref. 12,** p. 601)

284. D. Flunisolide is a steroid given by inhalation for management of bronchial asthma. The route of administration allows for less systemic effect when using glucocorticoids for anti-inflammatory treatment of asthma. (**Ref. 1,** pp. 291, 557; **Ref. 4,** pp. 1449, 1456; **Ref. 10,** pp. 1996–1997; **Ref. 12,** p. 601)

285. C. Dexamethasone and betamethasone are orally-effective glucocorticoids with a biologic half life of 3 to 4 days. (**Ref. 1,** p. 546; **Ref. 4,** p. 1447; **Ref. 12,** p. 596)

286. B. Prednisolone is prednisone with the 11-keto group reduced to a hydroxyl group. These compounds are used interchangeably. (**Ref. 4,** p. 1447)

287. B. Glipizide is an oral hypoglycemic agent that requires the presence of pancreatic beta cells for its action. It has approximately 100 times the potency of tolbutamide. (**Ref. 1,** p. 597; **Ref. 4,** pp. 1485–1486; **Ref. 10,** p. 2061; **Ref. 12,** p. 650)

288. D. The administration of glucagon causes hyperglycemia through hepatic glycolysis. It is used in the treatment of severe hypoglycemia in patients with diabetes mellitus. It is not effective in patients with chronic hypoglycemia or in hypoglycemia associated with starvation or adrenal insufficiency, because there is no liver store of glycogen in such patients. (**Ref. 1,** p. 599; **Ref. 4,** p. 1489; **Ref. 10,** p. 2075; **Ref. 12,** p. 652)

289. E. Ultralente insulin is a long-acting suspension of insulin in buffered water modified by the addition of zinc chloride. It is usually given as a single dose 30 to 60 minutes before breakfast. Patients previously using regular insulin should start with two-thirds of their total daily dose of regular insulin. (**Ref. 1,** pp. 589–590; **Ref. 4,** p. 1476; **Ref. 10,** p. 2047; **Ref. 12,** pp. 642–643)

290. A. The University Group Diabetes Program (UGDP) reported this still-unresolved adverse effect of tolbutamide in the early 1970s. Today package inserts still warn patients about the findings in this report. (**Ref. 1,** p. 596; **Ref. 4,** pp. 1486–1487; **Ref. 10,** p. 2071; **Ref. 12,** p. 649)

291. A. Androgen increases body hair, but has the potential to bring about patterns of male baldness when administered to females. (**Ref. 1,** pp. 578–579; **Ref. 4,** p. 1420)

292. C. Both androgen and estrogen bring about closure of the epiphyses. (**Ref. 1,** pp. 562, 578; **Ref. 4,** pp. 1386, 1416; **Ref. 12,** pp. 612, 628)

293. C. Both androgen and estrogen are synthesized, not only in the ovary, but in the testis as well. Fractionation of steroids contained in venous ovarian blood indicates that both testosterone and androstenedione, precursors of estrogens, are normal ovarian secretions. (**Ref. 1,** pp. 560, 568; **Ref. 4,** pp. 1387, 1416; **Ref. 12,** p. 628)

294. D. Although androgens do increase libido in hypogonadal men, they do not do so in normal men. Estrogens have a negative effect. (**Ref. 4,** p. 1424)

295. A. The more rapid action of T_3 may make it more useful in certain situations, such as hypothyroidism resulting from drug therapy or surgery, when a quicker action is needed. (**Ref. 1,** p. 534; **Ref. 4,** p. 1371; **Ref. 10,** p. 2104)

296. C. When T_4 is given in a dose four times greater than that of T_3, the elevation of metabolic rate produced by each is about equal and the effects of both continue after their disappearance from the blood. (**Ref. 4,** p. 1372; **Ref. 10,** p. 2099)

297. C. The largest source of natural estrogens is in the urine of a stallion. Liver, skeletal muscle, and other tissues also form estrogens. (**Ref. 1,** p. 560; **Ref. 3,** pp. 545–548; **Ref. 4,** p. 1385; **Ref. 12,** pp. 609–610)

298. D. Iodide administration can be used to reduce vascularity and cause the thyroid gland to become firm prior to surgery. Its onset of action occurs within 24 hours but it cannot suppress hyperthyroidism indefinitely. (**Ref. 1,** p. 536; **Ref. 4,** pp. 1377–1378; **Ref. 12,** p. 585)

299. C. The principal metabolite is hydroxyhexamide, which has a metabolic half-life that is considerably longer than the biologic half-life of the parent sulfonylurea drug. **(Ref. 1,** p. 597; **Ref. 3,** p. 569; **Ref. 4,** p. 1486; **Ref. 12,** p. 649)

300. B. The kidneys excrete chlorpropamide slowly, eliminating 80% to 90% of a single oral dose within 4 days. Usually 5 days of drug administration is required to reach a steady state, and up to 20 days are required for complete elimination if drug administration is stopped. **(Ref. 1,** p. 596; **Ref. 3,** p. 568; **Ref. 4,** p. 1486; **Ref. 12,** p. 649)

301. B. When glucose is given orally, greater amounts of insulin are secreted, apparently because of liberation of gastrin, secretin, pancreozymin, and "gut" glucagon. **(Ref. 1,** pp. 593–594; **Ref. 4,** p. 1466)

302. C. Although another form of iron for parenteral use is available in Europe, iron dextran is in general use in the United States at present. When specific indications for parenteral use of iron are present, the intravenous route is preferable to the intramuscular route because of the hazards or iron deposition in tissues. **(Ref. 1,** p. 454; **Ref. 3,** pp. 608–609; **Ref. 4,** p. 1292; **Ref. 12,** pp. 495–496)

303. A. Hemoglobin, which contains the major part, in combination with ferritin, holds the bulk of the total body iron. Trace amounts are found in myoglobin and heme-dependent and nonheme-dependent enzymes. **(Ref. 1,** p. 451; **Ref. 3,** p. 606; **Ref. 4,** p. 1283; **Ref. 12,** p. 493)

304. E. Vitamin B_{12} stores must be obtained from exogenous sources. The only natural source is microorganisms that grow in soil, sewage, and water. Once ingested, these organisms can live in the intestinal lumen and synthesize B_{12} for human use. **(Ref. 1,** p. 455; **Ref. 3,** p. 610; **Ref. 4,** pp. 1296–1297; **Ref. 12,** p. 497)

305. C. The only serious side effects associated with the use of erythropoietin are increased blood pressure and increased clotting in patients on dialysis machines. This is related to the increased volume of red cells and can be prevented by using lower doses, thus causing a more gradual increase in hematocrit. (**Ref. 1,** pp. 261–262; **Ref. 4,** p. 1281; **Ref. 12,** p. 504)

306. C. The process of hematopoiesis and lymphopoiesis (200 billion cells/day) is delicate; it is also a complex process involving networking and action at multiple steps, providing for synergistic interactions. (**Ref. 1,** pp. 461–462; **Ref. 4,** pp. 1278–1279; **Ref. 12,** pp. 504–505)

307. E. T-PA preferentially activates plasminogen bound to fibrin. This confines fibrinolysis to already-formed clots and lessens systemic effects. (**Ref. 1,** p. 471; **Ref. 3,** p. 465; **Ref. 4,** p. 1323; **Ref. 12,** p. 515)

308. D. Heparin is a mixture of mucopolysaccharides that act intravenously as anticoagulants. The activity is inhibited by the electropositive compound, protamine. Generally 1 mg protamine is given for every 100 units heparin remaining in the patient. (**Ref. 1,** pp. 467–468; **Ref. 3,** pp. 452, 454; **Ref. 4,** pp. 1313, 1317; **Ref. 12,** p. 511)

309. B. Folic acid corrects the megaloblastic anemia of B_{12} deficiency; however, the neurologic symptoms may progress. (**Ref. 3,** p. 614; **Ref. 4,** p. 1305)

310. A. Granulocyte/macrophage-colony stimulating factor will increase the proliferation of these cell lines in the bone marrow. (**Ref. 1,** p. 462; **Ref. 3,** p. 725; **Ref. 4,** p. 1282; **Ref. 12,** pp. 504–505)

311. C. Aspirin inhibits cyclooxygenase in platelets that cannot synthesize protein; hence, the TXA_2 production causing vasoconstriction is permanently inhibited. (**Ref. 1,** p. 472; **Ref. 3,** p. 459; **Ref. 4,** p. 1325; **Ref. 12,** p. 516)

312. B. Since heparin is effective in vitro it can be added to blood or placed in the blood to inhibit clot formation in and at sites where blood is passed through tubing or machines and/or where a cannula is in place. (**Ref. 1,** p. 467; **Ref. 3,** p. 454; **Ref. 4,** p. 1315; **Ref. 12,** p. 517)

313. B. The oral anticoagulants have no effect on the clotting factors that are already formed, but rather interfere with the action of vitamin K in the synthesis of factors II, VII, IX, and X. (**Ref. 1,** pp. 468–469; **Ref. 3,** pp. 455–456; **Ref. 4,** pp. 1317–1318; **Ref. 12,** p. 512)

314. A. In most instances, oral ferrous sulfate is the preferred treatment of iron-deficiency anemia, and it is relatively inexpensive. Since iron is absorbed in the upper small intestine, absorption of enteric-coated preparations is erratic. (**Ref. 1,** p. 453; **Ref. 3,** p. 608; **Ref. 4,** pp. 1289–1290; **Ref. 12,** p. 495)

315. B. In addition to the listed symptoms, riboflavin, or vitamin B$_2$, deficiency may produce anemia, which may be related to disturbances in folic acid metabolism. The physiologically-active forms of riboflavin, FMN and FAD, serve a vital role in metabolism as coenzymes for a wide variety of respiratory proteins. (**Ref. 3,** p. 617; **Ref. 4,** p. 1534)

316. C. All answers are true except that the fat-soluble vitamins are A, D, E, and K, whereas the water-soluble vitamins are the B-complex and C. (**Ref. 3,** pp. 615, 619; **Ref. 4,** pp. 1523–1524)

317. D. Vitamin A is necessary for differentiation and proliferation of epithelial cells. The lack of vitamin A leads to hyperplasia and a lack of differentiation. (**Ref. 3,** p. 620; **Ref. 4,** p. 1554)

318. C. There is no solid evidence that vitamin C (ascorbic acid) prevents the common cold; however, it does cause kidney stones, is high in fresh fruits and vegetables, and is necessary for collagen synthesis. (**Ref. 3,** p. 619; **Ref. 4,** pp. 1548–1550)

319. D. The disease rickets results from a lack of vitamin D. Scurvy is due to vitamin C deficiency. (**Ref. 1,** p. 611; **Ref. 3,** pp. 588, 619; **Ref. 4,** pp. 1510, 1514; **Ref. 12,** p. 664)

320. A. Renal stones may be caused by overdoses of vitamin C. Pyridoxine causes sensation changes. Nicotinic acid causes flushing, and a deficiency of vitamin K causes bleeding. Teratogenic effects can occur with large doses of vitamin A. (**Ref. 3,** p. 621; **Ref. 4,** pp. 1558–1559)

321. E. While there are several tocopherols, α-tocopherol is the most prevalent in animal tissues. It serves as an antioxidant. (**Ref. 3,** p. 621; **Ref. 4,** p. 1567)

322. E. Ultraviolet sunlight converts dietary 7-hydrocholesterol to the prohormone D_3 which is altered in the liver to 25-hydroxy D_3 and in the kidney to 1,25 dihydroxy D_3, which is bound to transport proteins in the blood. (**Ref. 3,** p. 586; **Ref. 4,** pp. 1511, 1515)

6

Drugs Acting on the Central Nervous System

GENERAL ANESTHETICS

DIRECTIONS (Questions 323–326): Each of the questions or incomplete statements below is followed by five suggested answers or completions. Select the **one** that is best in each case.

323. Given the following blood:gas partition coefficients, which of the following should be associated with the agent that induces anesthesia the most rapidly?
    A. 0.15
    B. 0.47
    C. 1.4
    D. 2.4
    E. 11

324. The halogenated anesthetic methoxyflurane
    A. has a potential of causing renal damage
    B. is flammable
    C. reduces uterine smooth muscle tone
    D. sensitizes the myocardium to catecholamines
    E. increases skeletal muscle tone

325. The sedative-hypnotic agent, diazepam, given intravenously, is used to induce anesthesia, and when compared with intravenous barbiturates
    A. gives a slower onset of anesthesia
    B. yields a longer postoperative period of amnesia
    C. tends to give light anesthesia
    D. has a shorter postoperative recovery period
    E. all of the above

326. All of the following are complications and undesirable features associated with the use of intravenous barbiturates EXCEPT
    A. danger of tissue necrosis from extravascular administration
    B. respiratory depression and apnea
    C. laryngospasm
    D. circulatory depression from overdose
    E. slow onset of action

DIRECTIONS (Questions 327–330): The group of questions below consists of five lettered headings followed by a list of numbered words, phrases, or statements. For each numbered word, phrase, or statement, select the **one** lettered heading that is most closely associated with it. Each lettered heading may be selected once, more than once, or not at all.

Questions 327–330:
    A. Halothane
    B. Enflurane
    C. Methoxyflurane
    D. Isoflurane
    E. Nitrous oxide

327. The most potent of the inhalation anesthetic agents

328. Seizures may occur during deep anesthesia with this agent, especially when hypocapnia is present

329. Unlike the other halogenated compounds listed above, myocardial function is well maintained during anesthesia with this agent

330. Only one of these five agents that does not decrease respiratory rate or tidal volume

DIRECTIONS (Questions 331–334): Each group of questions below consists of a diagram or table with three or four lettered components, followed by a list of numbered words, phrases, or statements. For each numbered word, phrase, or statement, select the **one** lettered component that is most closely associated with it. Each lettered component may be selected once, more than once, or not at all.

Questions 331–333 (Figure 8):

331. Brain, heart, and kidney

332. Skeletal muscle

333. Lung and blood

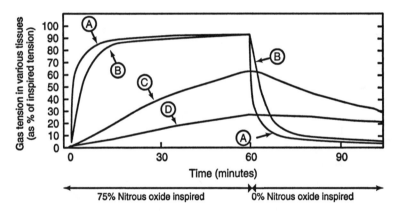

Figure 8 Tissue tensions of an anesthetic gas during uptake and elimination. (Adapted from Smith TC, Wollman H: History and principles of anesthesiology, in Gilman AG, Goodman LS, Rall TW, Murad F (Eds): *Goodman and Gilman's The Pharmacological Basis of Therapeutics,* 7th Ed. New York, Macmillan, 1985, p. 266, with permission.)

Question 334: Figure 9 shows distribution of thiopental in different body tissues and organs following its intravenous injection.

334. Skeletal muscle and skin

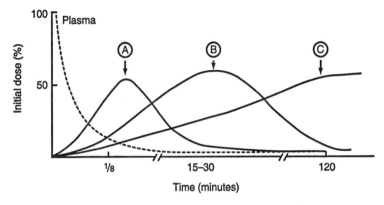

Figure 9 (Adapted from Price HL, et al: The uptake of thiopental by body tissues and its relation to the duration of narcosis. *Clin Pharmacol Ther* 1960; 1:16–22, with permission.)

DIRECTIONS (Questions 335–340): Each of the questions or incomplete statements below is followed by five suggested answers. Select the **one** that is best in each case.

---

335. The principal factor that determines the acceptability of an agent for use as a general anesthetic is
  A. rapid and pleasant induction of, and recovery from, anesthesia
  B. a wide margin of safety
  C. adequate relaxation of skeletal muscles
  D. the absence of adverse effects in the amount used
  E. analgesia

336. The ease with which the most widely-used inhalation anesthetics produce induction of anesthesia depends on all of the following EXCEPT
  A. a high blood:gas partition coefficient
  B. concentration of the anesthetic gas in the inspired air
  C. pulmonary ventilation
  D. transfer of anesthetic from alveoli to blood
  E. transfer of anesthetic gas from blood to tissue

337. The anesthetic agent halothane
  A. reduces stroke volume of the heart and systemic blood pressure
  B. stimulates the sympathetic nervous system
  C. slows the heart rate during anesthesia
  D. has an irritant effect on the tracheobronchial tree
  E. decreases catecholamine-induced arrhythmias

338. The intravenous anesthetic ketamine induces a state termed "dissociative anesthesia," which includes all of the following EXCEPT
  A. postanesthetic vivid dreams
  B. memory recall
  C. postanesthetic disorientation
  D. catatonia
  E. slight respiratory depression

339. The intravenous anesthetic thiopental
  A. is a potent depressant of respiration
  B. increases the respiratory response to increased plasma carbon dioxide
  C. increases intracranial pressure
  D. reversibly increases hepatic blood flow
  E. produces renal toxicity

340. Pharmacokinetic properties of an inhaled anesthetic include all of the following EXCEPT
  A. concentration of anesthetic inhaled
  B. solubility of anesthetic in the blood
  C. rate of pulmonary blood flow
  D. rate of anesthetic metabolism
  E. pulmonary ventilation

LOCAL ANESTHETICS

DIRECTIONS (Questions 341–345): Each of the questions or incomplete statements below is followed by five suggested answers or completions. Select the **one** that is best in each case.

341. The speed of nerve blockade by local anesthetics depends on all of the following factors EXCEPT
   A. whether neurons are myelinated or nonmyelinated
   B. whether neurons are small or large
   C. whether fibers are B or C or A type
   D. whether neurons are sensory or motor
   E. whether neurons conduct pain or tactile sensation

342. The central nervous system effects of intravenous local anesthetics are as follows EXCEPT
   A. light-headedness
   B. restlessness
   C. tremors
   D. irritability
   E. miosis

343. Each of the following statements is true for local anesthetics EXCEPT
   A. the ester type, such as procaine and tetracaine, is degraded principally by the liver
   B. the ester type is metabolized to p-aminobenzoic acid
   C. local anesthetics may cause asthmatic attacks in hypersensitive individuals
   D. allergic dermatitis has been reported
   E. allergic reactions are more likely to occur in the ester type than in the amide type

344. All of the following statements concerning local anesthetics are true EXCEPT
   A. increasing the calcium concentration to an isolated nerve potentiates the blocking action
   B. blockade results from preventing the elevated increase in the permeability of the excited membrane to sodium
   C. diazepam is the preferred drug for treating the convulsion caused by local anesthetics
   D. the ester type is hydrolyzed in the blood at a rapid rate
   E. drowsiness is the most common symptom of a CNS effect

345. Which of the following statements is true of cocaine?
  A. Its local vasoconstriction acts to limit its absorption, so that it can be applied to mucous membranes for surface anesthesia without systemic toxicity
  B. Its central stimulating action is manifested first in the medullary respiratory center
  C. It blocks both the excitatory and inhibitory responses of sympathetically-innervated organs to epinephrine, norepinephrine, and sympathetic nerve stimulation
  D. Its most important clinical action is its ability to block nerve conduction when applied topically; its most striking systemic effect is CNS stimulation
  E. It is not metabolized by the liver and depends on urinary excretion for its elimination from the body

---

DIRECTIONS (Questions 346–348): The group of questions below consists of five lettered headings followed by a list of numbered phrases or statements. For each numbered phrase or statement, select the one lettered heading that is most closely associated with it. Each lettered heading may be selected once, more than once, or not at all.

Questions 346–348:
  A. Tetracaine
  B. Prilocaine
  C. Mepivacaine
  D. Bupivacaine
  E. Etidocaine

346. A local anesthetic of the amide type, which may produce methemoglobinemia as a unique toxic after-effect

347. Long-acting derivative of lidocaine

348. A p-aminobenzoic acid ester producing a longer acting local anesthetic effect than that produced by procaine

SKELETAL MUSCLE RELAXANTS AND NEUROMUSCULAR-BLOCKING AGENTS

DIRECTIONS (Questions 349–352): Each of the words, questions, or incomplete statements below is followed by five suggested answers or completions. Select the one that is best in each case.

349. Succinylcholine
    A. may cause hypokalemia
    B. can be reversed by the administration of neostigmine during phase I
    C. is a depolarizing neuromuscular-blocking agent
    D. would be potentiated by tubocurarine
    E. is metabolized by the microsomal oxidase system

350. Tubocurarine
    A. produces fasciculations upon intravenous administration
    B. may lower blood pressure through histamine release
    C. has a prolonged duration of action in patients with an abnormal variant of pseudocholinesterase
    D. is utilized in the management of skeletal muscle spasticity
    E. augments the action of succinylcholine during phase I

351. Baclofen
    A. is superior to diazepam in relieving muscle spasm, since it causes less sedation
    B. is useful for producing flaccid paralysis prior to surgery
    C. should not be administered intrathecally due to its neurotoxicity
    D. is effectively antagonized by cholinesterase inhibitors
    E. is useful for managing malignant hyperthermia

352. All of the following statements concerning skeletal muscle relaxants are true EXCEPT
    A. skeletal muscle contraction is mediated by acetylcholine acting at nicotinic receptors
    B. aminoglycoside antibiotics may increase the neuromuscular blockade produced by tubocurarine
    C. succinylcholine may cause postoperative muscle pain

D. tubocurarine neuromuscular blockade would first be noted due to respiratory muscle paralysis

E. ventilation must be maintained in patients when neuromuscular blockers are administered

ANTICONVULSANTS

DIRECTIONS (Questions 353–356): Each of the questions or incomplete statements below is followed by five suggested answers or completions. Select the **one** that is best in each case.

353. Which of the following antiepileptic agents, used for trigeminal neuralgia, is considered a primary drug for the treatment of all seizure types except absence?
    A. Carbamazepine
    B. Ethosuximide
    C. Valproic acid
    D. Diazepam
    E. Phenobarbital

354. Which of the following anticonvulsants is most often used to treat absence (petit mal) seizures?
    A. Ethosuximide
    B. Phenobarbital
    C. Carbamazepine
    D. Bromide
    E. Diazepam

355. Most antiepileptic drugs act by
    A. dilation of blood vessels only at site of seizure focus
    B. constriction of blood vessels in the brain
    C. prevention of excessive discharge from seizure focus
    D. prevention of seizure spread into normal neurons
    E. increase in inhibitory impulses

356. Children who have experienced a convulsion associated with a
febrile illness have an increased risk of becoming epileptic. If anti-
convulsant therapy is indicated, the drug of choice is
  A. phenobarbital
  B. diazepam
  C. secobarbital
  D. phenytoin
  E. clonazepam

DIRECTIONS (Questions 357–360): The group of questions below
consists of five lettered headings followed by a list of numbered phrases or statements. For each numbered phrase or statement, select the **one**
lettered heading that is most closely associated with it. Each lettered
heading may be selected once, more than once, or not at all.

Questions 357–360:
  A. Valproic acid
  B. Primidone
  C. Phenytoin
  D. Diazepam
  E. Carbamazepine

357. An iminostilbene derivative structurally related to the tricyclic
antidepressants, which is particularly effective in treatment of partial seizures with complex symptomatology

358. Useful in treatment of absence seizures but has its greatest usefulness as a sole agent given intravenously for status epilepticus

359. First drug discovered that does not cause sedation and yet is effective in controlling epileptic seizures

360. A compound which is metabolized to a barbiturate

OPIOIDS

DIRECTIONS (Questions 361–376): Each of the questions or incomplete statements below is followed by five suggested answers or completions. Select the **one** that is best in each case.

---

361. All of the following are narcotics EXCEPT
   A. morphine
   B. codeine
   C. fentanyl
   D. meperidine
   E. diazepam

362. Each of the following is an action of morphine EXCEPT
   A. depression of the respiratory center
   B. adequate bioavailability when given orally
   C. release of histamine
   D. depression of the cough reflex
   E. tendency to dry secretions

363. Opioid analgesics include all of the following EXCEPT
   A. opiates derived from opium
   B. opiopeptides such as enkephalins
   C. synthetic compounds related to the opium alkaloids
   D. morphine
   E. ibuprofen

364. Each of the following statements is true concerning the nausea resulting from morphine administration EXCEPT
   A. it results from stimulation of the chemoreceptor trigger zone for emesis
   B. it occurs in approximately 40% of the ambulatory patients
   C. it is counteracted by morphine antagonists
   D. it is unique in that codeine in equianalgesic doses does not cause nausea
   E. it is partly due, in ambulatory patients, to an increase in vestibular sensitivity

365. All of the following substances are present in opium EXCEPT
   A. codeine
   B. thebaine
   C. morphine
   D. naloxone
   E. papaverine

366. All of the following are organ system effects of the narcotic analgesics EXCEPT
    A. euphoria
    B. respiratory depression
    C. emesis
    D. constipation
    E. myopia

367. Each of the following statements is true in relation to high biliary pressure caused in some patients by morphine EXCEPT
    A. results from spasm of the biliary tract
    B. results from increased tone of the sphincter of Oddi and is prevented by morphine antagonists
    C. is frequently accompanied by elevated serum lipase and serum amylase
    D. is completely relieved by atropine
    E. is relieved by opioid antagonists

368. Each of the findings listed is characteristic of opioid poisoning EXCEPT
    A. coma
    B. pinpoint pupils
    C. depressed respiration
    D. flaccidity of skeletal muscles
    E. elevated body temperature

369. In equianalgesic doses, methadone and morphine are similar in each of the following effects EXCEPT
    A analgesic potency
    B. antitussive action
    C. duration of analgesic action
    D. degree of respiratory depression
    E. miosis

370. Each of the following is an acceptable and satisfactory method for overcoming addiction to opioids EXCEPT
    A. administration of clonidine and methadone
    B. acute withdrawal
    C. a gradual daily reduction of the dose until no drug is being given

D. substituting methadone for morphine or heroin and then reducing the dose of methadone by 50% every other day

E. shifting the addict onto a methadone maintenance program

371. From 1 to 7 days after withdrawal of short-acting barbiturates, dependent individuals may manifest convulsions, hallucinations, and each of the following effects EXCEPT

A. vomiting
B. hypotension and tachycardia
C. fever
D. coarse tremors
E. sedation and sleepiness

372. Each of the following statements concerning the endogenous brain peptides with opiate-like activity is true EXCEPT

A. there is evidence for at least four types of receptors for these peptides and opioid drugs in the brain and other organs, designated mu, kappa, delta, and sigma
B. many synthetic congeners with preferential affinities for certain types of receptors have been prepared; these have been proved to be relatively selective agonists
C. three distinct families of these peptides, the enkephalins, the endorphins, and the dynorphins, are presently known to exist
D. each opioid family is derived from a genetically-distinct precursor polypeptide, which also contains a number of biologically-inactive peptides present exclusively in brain tissue
E. they appear to function as neurotransmitters, modulators of neurotransmission, or as neurohormones

373. Each of the following statements is true of meperidine, the prototype of the phenylpiperidine opioid analgesics, EXCEPT

A. many of the untoward effects of meperidine are caused by a metabolite, normeperidine
B. heart rate is not significantly affected by intramuscular administration, but intravenous doses often result in tachycardia
C. it differs from morphine in that toxic doses sometimes cause overt manifestations of CNS excitation
D. it has respiratory depressant actions that are not antagonized by naloxone
E. its adverse effects are similar to those occurring with equianalgesic doses of morphine except for less-frequent constipation and urinary retention

374. Morphine can be used in all of the following conditions EXCEPT
   A. cough
   B. acute pulmonary edema
   C. anesthetic premedication
   D. diarrhea
   E. for pain in patients with terminal cancer

375. Which of the following drugs may be used as a narcotic antagonist?
   A. Propoxyphene
   B. Fentanyl
   C. Naloxone
   D. Meperidine
   E. Naltrexone

376. The use of opioid analgesics may result in all of the following effects EXCEPT
   A. decrease in urine output
   B. tolerance
   C. decreased brain-stem response to carbon dioxide
   D. stimulates the release of antidiuretic hormone
   E. peripheral vasoconstriction

DIRECTIONS (Questions 377–386): Each group of questions below consists of five lettered headings followed by a list of numbered words, phrases, or statements. For each numbered word, phrase, or statement, select the **one** lettered heading that is most closely associated with it. Each lettered heading may be selected once, more than once, or not at all.

Questions 377–381:
   A. Pentazocine
   B. Dextromethorphan
   C. Diphenoxylate
   D. Propoxyphene
   E. Fentanyl

377. A preferred agent for treatment of diarrhea

378. The levo-isomer of this compound is an antitussive

379. A mixed agonist-antagonist

380. Short-acting opioid analgesic

381. An antitussive

Questions 382–386:
   A. Codeine
   B. Heroin
   C. Morphine-6-glucuronide
   D. Oxycodone
   E. Morphine-3-glucuronide

382. Used for nonproductive cough

383. Methylmorphine

384. An active metabolite of morphine

385. A morphine equivalent

386. An analgesic twice as potent as morphine

CENTRAL NERVOUS SYSTEM STIMULANTS

DIRECTIONS (Questions 387–392): The group of questions below consists of five lettered headings followed by a list of numbered phrases or statements. For each numbered phrase or statement, select the **one** lettered heading that is most closely associated with it. Each lettered heading may be selected once, more than once, or not at all.

Questions 387–392:
   A. Ephedrine
   B. Methylphenidate
   C. Theophylline
   D. Caffeine
   E. Cocaine

387. Side effects of this methylxanthine in treatment of asthma are nervousness and tremors

388. An orally-effective adrenergic amine

389. Used to treat children with attention-deficit hyperactivity disorder

390. Present in coffee at about 100 mg/cup

391. This widely abused nonadrenergic amine produces effects indistinguishable from those of amphetamine

392. Acts to increase catecholamines in the biophase by inhibiting transport

DRUGS AFFECTING BEHAVIOR

DIRECTIONS: Each of the questions or incomplete statements below is followed by five suggested answers or completions. Select the **one** that is best in each case.

393. The development of the current antipsychotic drugs is an outgrowth of research on
  A. atropine substitutes
  B. antianxiety drugs
  C. antihistamines
  D. sedative-hypnotic drugs
  E. antiemetics

394. Among the data supporting a role of dopamine antagonism in the therapeutic action of antipsychotic drugs are all of the following findings EXCEPT
  A. they increase the rate of production of dopamine metabolites in the midbrain
  B. small doses block behavioral and neuroendocrine effects of dopamine agonists
  C. they inhibit a dopamine-sensitive adenylate cyclase system in homogenates of caudate or limbic tissue
  D. inhibition of tyrosine hydroxylase, the rate-limiting enzyme in catecholamine biosynthesis, allows marked reduction of dose of these drugs in schizophrenic patients

E. drugs such as amphetamines, which block dopamine uptake at brain receptor sites, reduce symptoms of schizophrenia

395. Adverse effects of antipsychotic drugs include all of the following EXCEPT
  A. dry mouth
  B. Parkinson's syndrome
  C. infertility
  D. sinus arrhythmias
  E. drowsiness

396. The antipsychotic drugs are divided into the following chemical or drug classes EXCEPT
  A. heterocyclic compounds
  B. phenothiazines
  C. amphetamines
  D. thioxanthenes
  E. butyrophenones

397. The endocrine system is affected by the antipsychotic drugs leading to all of the following adverse effects EXCEPT
  A. gynecomastia in men
  B. amenorrhea
  C. dystonia
  D. galactorrhea
  E. false-positive pregnancy tests

DIRECTIONS (Questions 398–414): Each group of questions below consists of five lettered headings followed by a list of numbered words, phrases, or statements. For each numbered word, phrase, or statement, select the **one** lettered heading that is most closely associated with it. Each heading may be selected once, more than once, or not at all.

Questions 398–403:
  A. Loxapine
  B. Amoxapine
  C. Trazodone
  D. Molindone
  E. Haloperidol

398. An antidepressant agent chemically unrelated to tricyclic, tetra-cyclic, or other known antidepressant drugs

399. Representative of a new class of tricyclic antipsychotic agents chemically distinct from the thioxanthenes, butyrophenones, and phenothiazines

400. A dihydroindolone classified as an antipsychotic drug with a primary indication for treating schizophrenics

401. An antipsychotic drug that is very useful in situations where sedation and hypotension are undesirable

402. A second-generation antidepressant drug with a mild sedation component to its action

403. A butyrophenone antipsychotic drug with severe extrapyramidal adverse effects

Questions 404–408:
    A. Tranylcypromine
    B. Amitriptyline
    C. Thioridazine
    D. Clozapine
    E. Fluoxetine

404. Low incidence of extrapyramidal syndrome

405. May cause serious agranulocytosis

406. A tricyclic antidepressant drug

407. A monoamine oxidase (MAO) inhibitor used as an antidepressant drug

408. An antidepressant that specifically inhibits the uptake of serotonin

Questions 409–410:
    A. Clomipramine
    B. Isocarboxazid
    C. Imipramine

D. Methylphenidate
E. Lithium carbonate

409. Concomitant administration with a tricyclic antidepressant may result in increased plasma levels of the antidepressant

410. Tricyclic first-generation antidepressant drug

Questions 411–414:
    A. Tranylcypromine
    B. Meprobamate
    C. Chlordiazepoxide
    D. Chlorpromazine
    E. Mescaline

411. An anxiolytic drug found in combination products with anticholinergics, antidepressants and estrogen.

412. Possesses two modes of action: potent inhibition of monoamine oxidase and an amphetamine-like action

413. May produce postural hypotension, which has generally been attributed to an α-adrenergic blocking action

414. The occurrence of acute hypertensive crisis with fatal subarachnoid hemorrhage after ingestion of certain foods led to a curtailment of its use

---

DIRECTIONS (Questions 415–422): Each of the questions or incomplete statements below is followed by five suggested answers or completions. Select the **one** that is best in each case.

---

415. Chlorpromazine-related phenothiazine derivatives are useful therapeutic agents in the treatment of all of the following EXCEPT
    A. psychoses
    B. nausea and vomiting
    C. intractable hiccup
    D. motion sickness
    E. behavioral problems in children

416. The general characteristics of phenothiazines are that
   A. they seem to act by depressing the vomiting center rather than the trigger zone
   B. they possess α-adrenergic potentiating effects when given as a single dose
   C. they enhance the nicotinic and muscarinic actions of acetylcholine
   D. most of them possess significant antiemetic activity, making a wide choice of agents for this purpose possible
   E. they rarely cause drowsiness and are superior to other antipsychotic agents for this reason

417. The influence of phenothiazines on neuroendocrine activity
   A. is to inhibit release of growth hormone, perhaps by an action on the hypothalamus
   B. can be manifested as a delay in ovulation during chlorpromazine therapy, apparently as a result of the hypothalamus interfering with pituitary gonadotropin output
   C. may be manifested as amenorrhea, sometimes seen during therapy with large doses
   D. is to depress the hypothalamus, thereby interfering with milk formation in lactating patients by inhibiting release of lactogenic hormone
   E. may result in weight gain and increased appetite

418. Which of the following antipsychotics should not be used in diabetic or "prediabetic" patients:
   A. fluphenazine
   B. chlorpromazine
   C. haloperidol
   D. thioridazine
   E. chlorprothixene

419. All of the following statements concerning clozapine are true EXCEPT
   A. clozapine is considered an atypical antipsychotic because of its serotonergic, adrenergic, and cholinergic effects
   B. the most severe side-effect seen with this drug is a life threatening agranulocytosis
   C. clozapine raises the seizure threshold and may be useful in treating refractory seizures

D. unlike other antidepressants, clozapine has a limited effect on prolactin secretion

E. concurrent use with benzodiazepines has caused severe hypotension in some patients

420. The use of lithium carbonate in the treatment of bipolar affective disorder may lead to all of the following EXCEPT

A. tremor and other neurologic effects

B. weight loss

C. polydipsia and polyuria

D. altered T-wave leading to myocardial failure

E. edema

421. Benzodiazepines have all of the following effects EXCEPT

A. emetogenic

B. sedative-hypnotic

C. anticonvulsant

D. anxiolytic

E. muscle relaxant

422. The effects of benzodiazepines are believed to be mediated by which of the following neurotransmitters:

A. acetylcholine

B. glutethimide

C. γ-aminobutyric acid (GABA)

D. dopamine

E. serotonin

DIRECTIONS (Questions 423–427): Each group of questions below consists of five lettered headings followed by a list of numbered words, phrases, or statements. For each numbered word, phrase, or statement, select the one lettered heading that is most closely associated with it. Each heading may be selected only once.

A. Chloral hydrate

B. Temazepam

C. Meprobamate

D. Diazepam

E. Chlordiazepoxide

423. A benzodiazepine used in the treatment of insomnia

424. A benzodiazepine used in the treatment of acute alcohol withdrawal

425. A drug used in the emergency treatment of status epilepticus

426. A drug whose only approved use is as an anxiolytic and should not be used in patients with seizure disorders

427. A sedative particularly useful in children

DIRECTIONS: The incomplete statement below is followed by five suggested completions. Select the **one** that is best.

---

428. All of the following benzodiazepines are commonly used in the treatment of anxiety EXCEPT
   A. chlordiazepoxide
   B. clonazepam
   C. alprazolam
   D. lorazepam
   E. diazepam

DIRECTIONS (Questions 429–433): The group of questions below consists of five lettered headings followed by a list of numbered words, phrases, or statements. For each numbered word, phrase, or statement, select the one lettered heading that is most closely associated with it. Each heading may be selected only once.

   A. Fluoxetine
   B. Buspirone
   C. Phenobarbital
   D. Flumazenil
   E. Midazolam

429. An anxiolytic with very little sedating effect

430. A benzodiazepine antagonist

431. An antidepressant

432. A drug used for the purpose of inducing anterograde amnesia

433. A sedative-hypnotic also used in the treatment of epilepsy

---

DIRECTIONS (Questions 434–436): Each of the incomplete statements below is followed by five suggested completions. Select the **one** that is best in each case.

---

434. The earliest and longest lasting effect of lysergic acid diethylamide (LSD) is
  A. insomnia
  B. pupillary dilation
  C. hyperreflexia of the masseter muscles
  D. elevation of body temperature
  E. tachycardia with accompanying increase in blood pressure

435. All of the following statements concerning lithium blood levels are true EXCEPT
  A. they are monitored in order to establish a maintenance dose
  B. they are monitored to prevent toxicity
  C. they should be measured 10 to 12 hours following the last dose
  D. they are no longer required once a maintenance dose has been established
  E. initial levels should be taken approximately five days after treatment has been started

436. All of the following are side effects associated with the use of lithium EXCEPT
  A. anemia
  B. polydipsia
  C. tremor
  D. decreased thyroid function
  E. edema

DIRECTIONS (Questions 437–441): Each group of questions below consists of five lettered headings followed by a list of numbered words, phrases, or statements. For each numbered word, phrase, or statement, select the **one** lettered heading that is most closely associated with it. Each heading may be selected only once.

A. Ethchlorvynol
B. Estazolam
C. Sertraline
D. Flurazepam
E. Lithium

437. An antidepressant that acts primarily through the neurotransmitter serotonin

438. An older sedative-hypnotic agent

439. Signs of toxicity for this drug include profuse vomiting, diarrhea, and tremor

440. A benzodiazepine indicated only for use as a sedative-hypnotic

441. A benzodiazepine with a long half-life of approximately 50 to 100 hours

DIRECTIONS (Questions 442–444): Each of the questions or incomplete statements below is followed by five suggested answers or completions. Select the **one** that is best in each case.

442. In choosing a specific benzodiazepine for the treatment of insomnia, all of the following are considerations EXCEPT
A. age of the patient
B. mental status of the patient
C. the underlying sleep disorder being treated
D. the half-life of the drug
E. the absorption of the drug

443. All of the following increase the effects that the barbiturates have on the central nervous system EXCEPT
A. ethanol
B. antihistamines

C. isoniazid
D. steroids
E. monoamine oxidase inhibitors

444. All of the following statements concerning barbiturates are true EXCEPT
    A. they are used in the treatment of hypobilirubinemia in neonates
    B. absorption is increased if they are taken on an empty stomach
    C. they may cause paradoxical excitement in children
    D. they increase the effectiveness of oral contraceptives
    E. they increase the metabolism of coumarin anticoagulants

DIRECTIONS (Questions 445–449): Each group of questions below consists of five lettered headings followed by a list of numbered words, phrases, or statements. For each numbered word, phrase, or statement, select the **one** lettered heading that is most closely associated with it. Each heading may be selected only once.

    A. alprazolam
    B. amobarbital
    C. disulfiram
    D. thiopental
    E. chlorazepate

445. An ultra-short-acting barbiturate

446. A commonly used anxiolytic

447. A benzodiazepine used in the treatment of seizures

448. A long-acting barbiturate used as a sedative

449. Used in the treatment of alcoholism

DIRECTIONS (Questions 450–454): Each of the questions or incomplete statements below is followed by five suggested answers or completions. Select the **one** that is best in each case.

450. All of the following statements concerning ethanol are true EXCEPT
A. ethanol is a vasodilator
B. Wernicke-Korsakoff syndrome is associated with a deficiency in alcohol dehydrogenase
C. tolerance to the intoxicating effects of ethanol develops during continued use because of a change in metabolism
D. continued use of ethanol can result in anemia secondary to folate deficiencies
E. ethanol is metabolized primarily in the liver but also to a smaller extent by enzymes in the GI tract

451. Benzodiazepines are used in the treatment of all of the following EXCEPT
A. depression
B. insomnia
C. epilepsy
D. panic disorders
E. nausea and vomiting

452. Which of the following is a therapeutic use for ethanol?
A. sedation
B. induction of hepatic enzymes
C. reduction of anxiety
D. diuresis
E. injection for the relief of pain

453. The brief duration of action of the ultra-short-acting barbiturates is due to a
A. slow rate of excretion
B. high degree of protein binding
C. slow rate of metabolism in the liver
D. low lipid solubility, resulting in minimal concentration in the brain
E. rapid rate of redistribution from the brain due to increased lipid solubility

454. Ethanol has all of the following effects EXCEPT
A. diuretic effects on the kidney
B. increased blood concentration of catecholamines
C. decreased high-density lipoproteins
D. hepatic damage
E. teratogenic effects

DIRECTIONS (Questions 455–459): Each group of questions below consists of five lettered headings followed by a list of numbered words, phrases, or statements. For each numbered word, phrase, or statement, select the **one** lettered heading that is most closely associated with it. Each heading may be selected only once.

A. Midazolam
B. Paraldehyde
C. Pentobarbital
D. Phenobarbital
E. Oxazepam

455. A rapidly-acting sedative hypnotic

456. A short-acting barbiturate

457. Used in the treatment of seizures associated with tetanus

458. An active metabolite of chlorazepate

459. A benzodiazepine used primarily for preoperative sedation

DIRECTIONS (Questions 460–462): Each of the incomplete statements below is followed by five suggested completions. Select the **one** that is best in each case.

460. All of the following statements concerning benzodiazepines are true EXCEPT
   A. the majority of benzodiazepines are completely absorbed when taken orally
   B. mild dependence can develop following prolonged use
   C. flumazenil is an antagonist and can be used in cases of overdose
   D. benzodiazepines have no effect on REM sleep
   E. benzodiazepines have little or no effect on the cardiovascular system

461. Diazepam is used in the treatment of all of the following EXCEPT
   A. skeletal muscle spasms
   B. perioperative sedation
   C. status epilepticus
   D. anxiety
   E. analgesia

462. All of the following are associated with fetal alcohol syndrome EXCEPT
   A. impairment of growth
   B. a characteristic cluster of facial abnormalities
   C. extensive impairment of the immune system
   D. fatty infiltration of the liver and other hepatic disorders
   E. increased incidence of stillbirths and spontaneous abortions

Drugs Acting on the Central Nervous System

Answers and Discussion

323. A. In contrast to anesthetic agents with high partition coefficients, anesthetic agents with low partition coefficients are relatively insoluble gases that readily leave the blood and enter the brain, leading to a rapid induction of surgical anesthesia. (**Ref. 1,** p. 352; **Ref. 3,** pp. 379–380; **Ref. 4,** pp. 273, 286; **Ref. 12,** pp. 383–384)

324. A. Methoxyflurane is nonflammable, does not inhibit uterine smooth muscle tone, produces good skeletal muscle relaxation and does not sensitize the heart to catecholamines. Unfortunately, it stays in the body for a long period and is metabolized more than the other volatile agents. The production of fluorine ions is associated with renal toxicity. (**Ref. 1,** p. 355; **Ref. 3,** p. 392; **Ref. 4,** p. 297; **Ref. 12,** p. 389)

325. E. Diazepam is used to achieve anesthesia. Although the final depth of anesthesia is light, the recovery is slow and the patient will have a period of amnesia. (**Ref. 1,** pp. 359–360; **Ref. 4,** p. 304; **Ref. 12,** p. 391)

326. E. Intravenous barbiturates are useful for rapid induction or short procedures. They are contraindicated in patients with acute intermittent porphyria. **(Ref. 1,** p. 359; **Ref. 3,** p. 393; **Ref. 4,** p. 303; **Ref. 12,** p. 390)

327. C. Since the maximum allowable concentration (MAC) of methoxyflurane is only 0.16%, induction anesthesia can be achieved with inhaled concentrations of 2% to 3%; induction requires 20 to 30 minutes, however. Potency should not be confused with speed of induction. **(Ref. 1,** p. 377; **Ref. 4,** p. 285; **Ref. 12,** p. 387)

328. B. This excitatory action of enflurane is not thought to be of special concern, but the drug should be avoided in patients with seizure foci. **(Ref. 1,** p. 357; **Ref. 3,** p. 392; **Ref. 4,** p. 293; **Ref. 12,** p. 388)

329. D. Although blood pressure decreases with dose, cardiac output may increase markedly in response to hypercapnia with isoflurane anesthesia. **(Ref. 1,** p. 356; **Ref. 3,** p. 392; **Ref. 4,** p. 295; **Ref. 12,** p. 387)

330. E. Nitrous oxide is the one inhalation anesthetic that does not alter the heart or respiration when used with 15% to 20% oxygen. **(Ref. 1,** p. 357; **Ref. 3,** p. 391; **Ref. 4,** p. 299; **Ref. 12,** p. 388)

331. B. The brain, heart, and kidney are high blood-flow viscera to which significant amounts of anesthetic agents are delivered during administration, resulting in gas tension increases and decreases in these tissues paralleling those in blood. **(Ref. 1,** p. 354; **Ref. 3,** p. 380; **Ref. 4,** p. 275; **Ref. 12,** pp. 384–385)

332. C. Although the tissue:blood partition coefficient of most anesthetic agents is near unity for many lean body tissues, the blood flow to muscle is relatively low, so that equilibration of blood and tissue tensions is reached rather slowly. **(Ref. 1,** p. 354; **Ref. 3,** p. 380; **Ref. 4,** p. 275; **Ref. 12,** pp. 384–385)

333. A. With the first breath of anesthetic gas, the alveolar tension of nitrous oxide begins to increase and continues rapidly through the early uptake phase; the arterial tension of this gas reaches 90% of the inspired tension in about 20 minutes. The relatively poor blood flow to adipose tissue results in a slow increase in nitrous oxide gas tension in fat, but because of the high tissue: blood coefficient for these tissues, its concentration in fatty tissue is much greater than that in blood at the time of equilibrium. (**Ref. 1,** p. 354; **Ref. 3,** pp. 380–381; **Ref. 4,** pp. 275, 298; **Ref. 12,** pp. 384–385)

334. **B.** Following initial distribution of thiopental to brain and other tissues with high blood flow, a relatively rapid redistribution of the drug occurs, principally to "indifferent" tissues with a large mass, such as muscle. Although thiopental penetrates all cells readily, it has an especially high affinity for fat. The delay in the peak concentration observed in curve C is due to the relatively poor blood supply to this tissue. The rapid entry of thiopental into the brain, liver, and kidneys is related to its high lipid solubility, and the short duration of the resulting anesthesia to its redistribution from the brain, which it leaves rapidly. (**Ref. 1,** p. 359; **Ref. 3,** p. 393; **Ref. 4,** p. 302; **Ref. 12,** p. 390)

335. **D.** Although all of these are characteristics of an ideal anesthetic agent, rapid induction may be achieved by use of ultra-short-acting barbiturates, analgesia by opioids, and specific muscle relaxants may be used to relax skeletal muscle. With the newer agents now employed, safety has become less of an issue. The incidence of adverse effects now governs selection, even though it may be argued that this is a safety issue. (**Ref. 1,** p. 350; **Ref. 3,** pp. 376–377; **Ref. 4,** p. 285; **Ref. 12,** p. 331)

336. **A.** Ease of administration and rapidity of induction depends on all factors listed except a high lipid solubility as indicated by a high blood gas partition coefficient. The more soluble an agent the slower will be the induction time. (**Ref. 1,** p. 352; **Ref. 4,** pp. 271–273; **Ref. 12,** pp. 383–384)

337. **A.** Halothane depresses the heart and circulation, but does not evoke a compensatory increase in sympathetic nervous system activity. It does not usually produce respiratory depression. (**Ref. 1,** p. 356; **Ref. 3,** pp. 394–395; **Ref. 4,** p. 307; **Ref. 12,** pp. 387–388)

338. **B.** Recovery from ketamine anesthesia can result in the "dissociative" state, and this has limited the use of this drug. However, the amnesia has some advantages. Ketamine is used for short

anesthesia. It does not produce renal toxicity, nor does it increase intracranial pressure. (**Ref. 1,** p. 360; **Ref. 3,** pp. 393–394; **Ref. 4,** p. 306; **Ref. 12,** p. 392)

339. A. Thiopental is commonly used for short surgical procedures. It is also used to induce anesthesia. Due to respiratory and cardiovascular depression, this agent is not often used as the sole anesthetic for general anesthesia. (**Ref. 1,** p. 359; **Ref. 2,** pp. 473–474; **Ref. 8,** p. 303; **Ref. 9,** p. 423; **Ref. 12,** p. 390)

340. D. The inhaled anesthetics are metabolized to such a minor extent that this factor is not used in establishing the pharmacokinetic properties of these agents. (**Ref. 1,** pp. 352–354; **Ref. 3,** p. 381; **Ref. 4,** pp. 273–274; **Ref. 12,** pp. 383–386)

341. D. There are general patterns of loss of nerve conduction observed with local anesthetic agents. If categorization is based on myelination, frequency, size, or fiber type, then unmyelinated fibers, rapidly depolarizing (ie, pain), small fibers, and C fibers are blocked before myelinated fibers, fibers with slow firing rates, large fibers, or A and B fibers. There is no distinction between motor and sensory function. However, there is overlap between these categories. (**Ref. 1,** pp. 366–367; **Ref. 3,** p. 399; **Ref. 4,** pp. 313–314, 316; **Ref. 12,** pp. 398–399)

342. E. Local anesthetics are administered in such a way as to avoid tonic-clonic convulsions that result from high blood levels. The early signs of toxicity include light-headedness, restlessness, shivers, irritability, and rapid eye movements. With infiltration anesthesia, epinephrine may be added to reduce absorption of the local anesthetic; however, it should not be added where there are end arteries, such as in fingers, toes, ears, nose, and penis. (**Ref. 1,** p. 368; **Ref. 3,** p. 401; **Ref. 4,** p. 317; **Ref. 12,** p. 401)

343. A. The plasma pseudocholinesterase is mostly responsible for degrading the ester type of local anesthetics, though the liver contributes. The liberated products, especially PABA, have been implicated in the occasional allergic reactions. (**Ref. 1,** pp. 365, 369; **Ref. 3,** pp. 399–401; **Ref. 4,** pp. 318–319; **Ref. 12,** pp. 397, 402)

344. A. The degree of blockade is reduced, not increased, as calcium levels are increased. Local anesthetics act by their direct interaction with voltage-sensitive Na^+ channels. (**Ref. 1**, pp. 365–366; **Ref. 4**, p. 312; **Ref. 12**, p. 398)

345. D. The marked stimulation, particularly of the cerebral cortex, by cocaine, even when applied topically, has led to limited use even for topical anesthesia. Other effective and less toxic drugs are now available. Effects of adrenergic amines on sympathetically-innervated organs are potentiated. (**Ref. 1**, pp. 367–368; **Ref. 3**, pp. 401–402; **Ref. 4**, p. 319)

346. B. Prilocaine has pharmacologic properties similar to those of lidocaine, but has a longer onset and duration of action. (**Ref. 1**, pp. 364, 369; **Ref. 4**, p. 321; **Ref. 12**, pp. 401–402)

347. E. The time required for production of anesthesia with etidocaine is about the same as for lidocaine, but its anesthetic action lasts two to three times longer. (**Ref. 1**, p. 364; **Ref. 4**, p. 320; **Ref. 12**, p. 398)

348. A. Tetracaine is about 10 times more toxic and more active than procaine. (**Ref. 1**, p. 364; **Ref. 3**, p. 403; **Ref. 4**, p. 321; **Ref. 12**, p. 396)

349. C. The depolarizing skeletal-muscle blocking agent, succinylcholine, has a short duration of action due to rapid hydrolysis by plasma cholinesterases. It has the potential to cause hyperkalemia, especially in burn patients. Tubocurarine antagonizes succinylcholine, and inhibition of cholinesterase would potentiate the blockade if administered during phase I. (**Ref. 1**, pp. 374–375, 378; **Ref. 3**, pp. 133–134; **Ref. 4**, pp. 171–172, 176; **Ref. 12**, pp. 409, 413)

350. B. Tubocurarine is the neuromuscular blocking agent most apt to cause histamine release. It causes a flaccid paralysis, in contrast to the fasciculations seen with succinylcholine. It is succinylcholine that has a prolonged action with genetic variants of pseudocholinesterase. Tubocurarine is of no use for skeletal muscle spasticity, and it would antagonize succinylcholine during phase I.

(**Ref. 1,** pp. 375, 377–378; **Ref. 3,** pp. 129–131; **Ref. 4,** pp. 172, 174; **Ref. 12,** p. 412)

351. A. Diazepam is employed for muscle spasms, however sedation limits its usefulness in many patients. Flaccid paralysis is obtained by intravenous administration of tubocurarine. Baclofen is utilized for muscle spasticity and while it is effective orally, recent studies have shown that intrathecal administration may prove effective for long-term therapy. Cholinesterase inhibitors that penetrate centrally, such as physostigmine, provide questionable usefulness. Dantrolene is the agent of choice to interfere with excitation-contraction coupling in malignant hypothermia. (**Ref. 1,** pp. 380–381; **Ref. 3,** pp. 134–137; **Ref. 4,** pp. 479–480; **Ref. 12,** pp. 415–416)

352. D. Muscle paralysis follows the pattern of jaw and eye movement, larger limb muscles, and lastly the intercostal muscles and then the diaphragm. Recovery is in the reverse order. (**Ref. 1,** pp. 372, 376, 378; **Ref. 3,** pp. 129, 131; **Ref. 4,** pp. 166, 173, 175, 176; **Ref. 12,** pp. 410, 412)

353. A. Carbamazepine was first used to treat trigeminal neuralgia. It is now considered a primary choice for generalized seizures and simple partial seizures. It is not used for absence seizures. (**Ref. 1,** p. 336; **Ref. 4,** pp. 447, 449, 458; **Ref. 12,** pp. 365–366)

354. A. For generalized seizures of the absence type characterized by 3/sec spike-and-wave EEG patterns, ethosuximide, valproic acid, and clonazepam are used. Valproic acid, in spite of a possible hepatotoxic effect, is considered equal to ethosuximide and superior to it if tonic-clonic seizures emerge. It is difficult to establish the correct dosage of clonazepam. (**Ref. 1,** pp. 339, 341, 343; **Ref. 4,** p. 458; **Ref. 12,** p. 371)

355. D. Antiepileptic drugs have effects on sodium conduction, potassium channels, calcium channels, GABA, and a variety of other systems. However, it is generally accepted that these agents act through a reduction in the likelihood that the excessive discharges will spread over normal neurons. (**Ref. 1,** pp. 337–338; **Ref. 4,** p. 438; **Ref. 12,** pp. 361–362)

356. A. Although it is questionable whether all children who have had a seizure should receive any treatment, those at highest risk may profit by chronic therapy with phenobarbital. (**Ref. 1,** p. 338; **Ref. 4,** p. 458; **Ref. 12,** p. 368)

357. E. Carbamazepine, like phenytoin, is effective in relieving generalized tonic-clonic seizures, but is ineffective in absence seizures and might make these seizures worse. (**Ref. 1,** pp. 336–337; **Ref. 4,** pp. 447, 449; **Ref. 12,** pp. 366–367)

358. D. Diazepam is a benzodiazepine used for status epilepticus. Lorazepam, which has a longer duration of action, is preferred by some physicians. (**Ref. 1,** p. 347; **Ref. 4,** p. 459; **Ref. 12,** p. 374)

359. C. Phenytoin, in adequate but minimal effective doses, usually does not cause sedation. (**Ref. 1,** p. 333; **Ref. 4,** p. 440; **Ref. 12,** p. 365)

360. B. Primidone is not a barbiturate, even though it is classed with this group of agents. It is metabolized to phenobarbital and phenylethylmalonamide, both of which have antiepileptic activity. (**Ref. 12,** pp. 368–369)

361. E. There are at least 17 commonly-used opioid agents. These include morphine, codeine, fentanyl, and meperidine. The hypnotic-sedative diazepam is not an opioid. (**Ref. 1,** pp. 310, 423; **Ref. 4,** pp. 486, 490; **Ref. 12,** pp. 374, 461–462)

362. B. All of these effects on the respiratory system make it advisable not to use morphine and related drugs during an asthmatic episode. The bioavailability due to first pass metabolism after absorption from the gastrointestinal tract varies among drugs; methadone, for example, is much more completely absorbed. Adequate analgesia can be obtained if the oral/parenteral effectiveness ratios are considered in dosing. (**Ref. 1,** pp. 426, 427; **Ref. 4,** pp. 493, 496, 497, 499; **Ref. 5,** p. 97; **Ref. 6,** p. 2071; **Ref. 12,** pp. 463, 467)

363. E. Whereas the term opioid analgesics includes the products from opium and the somewhat chemically related narcotics, the term now includes the opiopeptins, such as enkephalin. (**Ref. 1,** p. 420; **Ref. 4,** p. 486; **Ref. 5,** p. 95; **Ref. 12,** pp. 460–462)

364. D. In the recumbent position, nausea after morphine administration is markedly less common; codeine shares with morphine the side effect of causing nausea and vomiting in some patients. (**Ref. 1,** p. 427; **Ref. 4,** p. 493; **Ref. 12,** p. 468)

365. D. More than 20 alkaloids have been identified as constituents of opium, but only three are important in therapeutics, ie, morphine, codeine, and papaverine. (**Ref. 1,** p. 420; **Ref. 4,** p. 489)

366. E. Emesis, constipation, and respiratory depression are the common effects of the narcotics. Some patients experience euphoria. Myopia has to do with vision; miosis, or pinpoint pupils, is an effect of the narcotics. (**Ref. 1,** pp. 426, 427; **Ref. 4,** pp. 492–494; **Ref. 12,** pp. 467–468)

367. D. Although morphine reduces bile formation, the obstruction to its outflow elevates the bile pressure, causing distension of ducts within the liver (true for pancreatic juice and the pancreas also), and causing amylase and lipase to pass into the bloodstream. Atropine only partially relieves the spasm. (**Ref. 1,** pp. 427, 434; **Ref. 4,** pp. 495; **Ref. 12,** p. 468)

368. E. The three findings—coma, pinpoint pupils, and depressed respiration—are known as the triad typical of acute opioid poisoning. Body temperature is reduced, resulting in a cold, clammy skin. (**Ref. 4,** p. 500)

369. C. Although morphine and methadone are quite similar in many respects, methadone does differ in that it is well absorbed following oral administration and it has a 24-hour half-life making its duration longer. These properties make it useful in treating heroin abusers. (**Ref. 3,** p. 329; **Ref. 4,** pp. 508–509)

370. B. Sudden withdrawal from an addictive drug is definitely inadvisable and may be life-threatening. Methadone substitution is one of the acceptable methods. (**Ref. 1,** pp. 438, 439; **Ref. 3,** pp. 339–340; **Ref. 4,** pp. 508, 509; **Ref. 12,** p. 480)

371. E. The intensity and duration of the symptoms are influenced by the degree of barbiturate dependence. Convulsions have occurred up to 7 days after withdrawal. (**Ref. 1**, pp. 439–440; **Ref. 3**, p. 342; **Ref. 4**, pp. 561–562; **Ref. 12**, p. 481)

372. D. Each precursor contains several biologically-active opioids and nonopioid peptides that have been detected in blood and various tissues. (**Ref. 1**, pp. 424–425; **Ref. 4**, pp. 486–487; **Ref. 12**, pp. 464–465)

373. D. The respiratory depression produced by meperidine is equal to that seen with equianalgesic doses of morphine. This, along with the sedative effects, is rapidly antagonized by naloxone and other opioid antagonists. (**Ref. 3**, pp. 327–328; **Ref. 4**, pp. 504–506)

374. A. Morphine will suppress cough; however, codeine or preferably dextromethorphan should be used. One of the early uses of morphine and opium extracts was to treat diarrhea. However, synthetic compounds with almost no dependence liability are now available. Most morphine addicts suffer from chronic constipation. (**Ref. 1**, pp. 428–429; **Ref. 4**, pp. 501–504; **Ref. 12**, p. 474)

375. C. Naloxone is nearly a pure antagonist for morphine and the opioids. Given intravenously, it will quickly overcome the depressant effects of the opioids. Naltrexone is a long-acting antagonist used to assist opioid abusers in remaining drug free. (**Ref. 1**, p. 434; **Ref. 3**, pp. 330–331; **Ref. 4**, p. 517; **Ref. 12**, pp. 474–475)

376. E. Opioid analgesics have a wide range of effects. Tolerance is well recognized, as is constipation. However, the neuroendocrine effects are often overlooked. Histamine release causes vasodilation and pruritus, rather than vasoconstriction. (**Ref. 1**, pp. 427–428; **Ref. 3**, pp. 324–325; **Ref. 4**, pp. 492–493; **Ref. 12**, p. 468)

377. C. Diphenoxylate usually comes in combination with atropine sulfate. The compound has no morphine-like subjective effects following a single dose, but repeated administration produces typical opioid activity. (**Ref. 1**, p. 433; **Ref. 3**, p. 329; **Ref. 4**, p. 507; **Ref. 5**, p. 927; **Ref. 12**, pp. 473–474)

378. D. Dextropropoxyphene has opioid-like activity. The levo-isomer is used as a centrally-acting antitussive. Propoxyphene in the low 32 mg dose combined with aspirin has little more analgesic activity than aspirin alone. (**Ref. 1**, p. 432; **Ref. 3**, p. 333; **Ref. 4**, pp. 507, 518; **Ref. 5**, p. 108; **Ref. 12**, p. 474)

379. A. Pentazocine was developed as a compound with analgesic activity that has low abuse potential. However, tolerance develops and withdrawal occurs. The concept of a competitive antagonist at mu receptors with agonist activity at kappa receptors making it nonaddicting has yet to be realized. (**Ref. 1**, p. 433; **Ref. 3**, p. 331; **Ref. 4**, p. 510, 512; **Ref. 5**, p. 109; **Ref. 12**, p. 474)

380. E. The compound fentanyl is a mu agonist with a potency 80 times that of morphine. It can be used alone but is often combined with droperidol. (**Ref. 1**, p. 423, **Ref. 3**, p. 328; **Ref. 4**, p. 508; **Ref. 5**, p. 469; **Ref. 12**, pp. 463, 473)

381. B. Dextromethorphan has no analgesic or addictive properties. It is widely used in over-the-counter cough medications. (**Ref. 1**, p. 433; **Ref. 3**, p. 333; **Ref. 4**, p. 518; **Ref. 5**, p. 469; **Ref. 12**, p. 474)

382. A. Codeine is widely used in combination products, including nonopioid analgesics, and as an antitussive in cough syrups. It should not be given to individuals with productive cough, since secretions are removed by coughing. (**Ref. 3**, p. 333; **Ref. 4**, p. 500; **Ref. 5**, p. 468; **Ref. 12**, p. 474)

383. A. Morphine can be formed by demethylating codeine. Codeine, which has a low affinity for mu receptors, has analgesic action due to conversion to morphine. Heroin is diacetyl morphine. It is also converted to morphine in the body. (**Ref. 3**, p. 327; **Ref. 4**, pp. 498, 500; **Ref. 12**, p. 461)

384. C. Morphine is conjugated at both the 3 and 6 position. The main route of metabolism is to an inactive 3-glucuronide. However, the 6-glucuronide is more potent than morphine. In patients with renal failure, toxicity may result due to accumulation of the active metabolite. (**Ref. 1**, p. 425; **Ref. 3**, p. 325; **Ref. 4**, p. 497; **Ref. 5**, p. 103; **Ref. 12**, p. 464)

385. D. Oxycodone is about the same as morphine in potency but it has a greater oral effectiveness with an oral/parenteral ratio of approximately 2. The ratio for morphine is 6. Oxycodone is often combined with aspirin or acetaminophen. (**Ref. 1**, p. 432; **Ref. 4**, p. 500; **Ref. 5**, pp. 96, 105; **Ref. 12**, p. 463)

386. B. Diacetylmorphine (heroin) is not available for therapeutic use in the United States. It is twice as potent as morphine but has no unique therapeutic advantages despite claims to the contrary. It has a much higher abuse potential. (**Ref. 1**, p. 432; **Ref. 3**, p. 327; **Ref. 4**, p. 500; **Ref. 12**, p. 473)

387. C. Theophylline and aminophylline are used to treat chronic asthma. The use of these compounds has decreased due to emphasis on treating the inflammatory component of the disease. Major side effects are nervousness and tremors. Increased doses can lead to restlessness, agitation, emesis, and tachycardia. (**Ref. 1**, pp. 284–285; **Ref. 4**, p. 628; **Ref. 12**, pp. 310–311)

388. A. Ephedrine is an orally-effective adrenergic amine that stimulates β_2-adrenergic receptors. The use of selective agents that cause less cardiac stimulation and less CNS stimulation have caused it to be used less frequently. (**Ref. 1**, p. 286; **Ref. 4**, p. 214; **Ref. 12**, p. 125)

389. B. Double-blind studies with placebo control have demonstrated that methylphenidate can improve both behavior and learning ability in 50% to 75% of these children, although indiscriminate use in such children is not approved. (**Ref. 1**, p. 212; **Ref. 4**, p. 217; **Ref. 12**, p. 129)

390. D. Caffeine is present in coffee and tea. Depending on how the coffee is made, a cup contains about 100 mg of caffeine. Patients are often warned about the use of coffee before certain medical procedures. Caffeine may also be used to manage apnea of preterm infants. (**Ref. 1**, pp. 440–441; **Ref. 4**, pp. 628–630; **Ref. 12**, pp. 481–482)

391. E. Cocaine when injected intravenously produces subjective effects that are almost indistinguishable from those of dextroamphetamine. It is not uncommon to refer to cocaine as "super-speed". Amphetamine is "speed." (**Ref. 1,** p. 442; **Ref. 4,** p. 540; **Ref. 12,** p. 483)

392. **E.** Cocaine inhibits the membrane transporter and it is referred to as an inhibitor of membrane uptake. Ephedrine releases catecholamines and methylphenidate acts in a similar manner. The methylxanthine compounds most likely act at postreceptor sites to increase the second messenger, since they are inhibitors of phosphodiesterase. (**Ref. 1,** p. 441; **Ref. 4,** pp. 191, 213, 623; **Ref. 12,** p. 482)

393. **C.** The prototype of the phenothiazine drugs, chlorpromazine, was developed as an antihistamine, but was observed to have a beneficial effect in psychotic patients, thus leading to the introduction of a large number of related compounds for their antipsychotic activity. (**Ref. 1,** p. 395; **Ref. 3,** p. 242; **Ref. 4,** p. 386; **Ref. 12,** p. 432)

394. **E.** Amphetamines are known to release dopamine in the brain and can exacerbate schizophrenic symptoms, which are blocked by dopamine antagonists such as chlorpromazine. (**Ref. 1,** p. 395; **Ref. 3,** pp. 242–243; **Ref. 4,** p. 390; **Ref. 12,** pp. 435–436)

395. **D.** The antipsychotic drugs are not used by addicts. They complain of how unpleasant the drugs make them feel. Antipsychotics produce a depressed feeling, urinary retention, and dry mouth. These agents cause hyperprolactinemia, leading to amenorrhea, galactorrhea, and infertility. (**Ref. 1,** pp. 402–403; **Ref. 3,** pp. 244–248; **Ref. 4,** pp. 395, 398; **Ref. 12,** pp. 439–441)

396. **C.** The early antipsychotic drugs were derivatives of phenothiazine. The thioxanthene compounds are related to the phenothiazines. The butyrophenones, dihydroindolones, and dibenzoxazepines are not chemically related to the earlier antipsychotic drugs. (**Ref. 1,** p. 396; **Ref. 3,** p. 242; **Ref. 4,** p. 386; **Ref. 12,** pp. 432–433)

397. **C.** The antipsychotics produce marked endocrine changes such as hyperprolactinemia. These effects include amenorrhea, galactorrhea, impotence, and decreased libido. (**Ref. 1,** p. 399; **Ref. 3,** p. 248; **Ref. 4,** pp. 392–393; **Ref. 12,** p. 437)

398. C. Trazodone is thought to exert its antidepressant effects by inhibiting the reuptake of norepinephrine and serotonin. Its long acting metabolite, m-chlorophenyl piperazine, stimulates serotonin receptors. (**Ref. 1,** p. 410; **Ref. 3,** p. 260; **Ref. 4,** p. 406; **Ref. 12,** pp. 451–452)

399. A. Most of loxapine's effects on the CNS resemble those produced by the phenothiazines, although it appears less likely to cause sedation, weight gain, and extrapyramidal symptoms. (**Ref. 1,** p. 401; **Ref. 3,** p. 250; **Ref. 4,** p. 397; **Ref. 6,** p. 1781; **Ref. 12,** p. 438)

400. D. Molindone produces moderate sedation, increased activity, and possibly euphoria without causing muscle relaxation or incoordination, apparently through an action on the reticular activating system. (**Ref. 1,** p. 401; **Ref. 3,** p. 250; **Ref. 4,** p. 397; **Ref. 6,** p. 1949; **Ref. 12,** p. 438)

401. E. Haloperidol has less-prominent tranquilizing properties than does chlorpromazine, although it shares the prominent side-effect of production of extrapyramidal syndromes. Haloperidol is also useful in the treatment of certain severe behavior problems in children. (**Ref. 3,** p. 250; **Ref. 4,** p. 397; **Ref. 6,** p. 1489; **Ref. 10,** p. 1443; **Ref. 12,** p. 438)

402. B. Amoxapine is of the same chemical class as loxapine, but is indicated for the relief of symptoms of depression in patients with certain neurotic and psychotic disorders, and thus is classified as an antidepressant, rather than an antipsychotic drug. (**Ref. 3,** pp. 258–259; **Ref. 6,** p. 269; **Ref. 10,** pp. 1388–1389; **Ref. 12,** p. 454)

403. E. Haloperidol is a butyrophenone with the disadvantage of possible severe extrapyramidal syndrome. (**Ref. 3,** p. 250; **Ref. 4,** p. 397; **Ref. 6,** p. 1489; **Ref. 10,** p. 1443; **Ref. 12,** p. 438)

404. C. Thioridazine is an antipsychotic phenothiazine with a low incidence of extrapyramidal syndrome. (**Ref. 4,** p. 396; **Ref. 6,** p. 2214)

405. D. Clozapine is a dibenzodiazepine antipsychotic drug with few side effects except a reported 3% incidence of severe agranulocytosis. For this reason, patients must be monitored at weekly intervals. (**Ref. 1,** p. 403; **Ref. 4,** p. 401; **Ref. 6,** p. 876; **Ref. 10,** p. 1434; **Ref. 12,** p. 440)

406. **B.** Amitriptyline is a prototype drug of the tricyclic class and it is a commonly used antidepressant with some sedative action. (**Ref. 1,** p. 413; **Ref. 3,** p. 258; **Ref. 4,** p. 411; **Ref. 12,** p. 449)

407. **A.** The MAO inhibitors, such as tranylcypromine, isocarboxazid, and phenelzine, have been used to treat unusual depressions such as hypochondria and phobias. (**Ref. 1,** p. 412; **Ref. 3,** p. 258; **Ref. 4,** pp. 414–415; **Ref. 12,** pp. 450–451)

408. **E.** Fluoxetine is a unique antidepressant in that it acts almost solely through the blockade of serotonin reuptake. For this reason, many of the side effects seen with other agents are eliminated. (**Ref. 1,** pp. 410–411; **Ref. 3,** p. 237; **Ref. 12,** p. 451)

409. **D.** Potentiation of the effects of tricyclic drugs by methylphenidate can result from interference with their metabolism in the liver. This also occurs when tricyclics are given with neuroleptic drugs and certain steroids, including oral contraceptives. (**Ref. 4,** p. 413; **Ref. 6,** p. 265; **Ref. 10,** p. 1387)

410. **C.** Imipramine and amitriptyline are the first of the tricyclic antidepressants to be developed. Imipramine is metabolized to an active metabolite, desipramine, which has been used independently as an antidepressant. (**Ref. 1,** p. 410; **Ref. 3,** p. 254; **Ref. 4,** p. 405; **Ref. 12,** p. 451)

411. **C.** Chlordiazepoxide is available as a combination product with an anticholinergic (clidinium), an antidepressant (amitriptyline), and with estrogen. It is recommended that therapy be initiated with each individual agent in order to determine appropriate doses before a combination product is selected. (**Ref. 10,** p. 1495)

412. **A.** The rapid onset and behavioral effects produced by tranylcypromine are consequences of its amphetamine-like action, and its sustained antidepressant effects are related to the inhibition of MAO. (**Ref. 4,** p. 415; **Ref. 10,** p. 1382)

413. D. Intravenous administration of chlorpromazine in normal men causes orthostatic hypotension due to a combination of central effects, peripheral α-adrenergic blockade, and reflex tachycardia. Oral administration produces considerably less hypotension, to which the body generally adapts over time. (**Ref. 4,** pp. 393, 396; **Ref. 10,** p. 1411)

414. A. The ingestion by patients on tranylcypromine of certain foods containing tyramine or other monoamines normally detoxified by MAO causes severe hypertensive episodes. Patients should be counseled to avoid cheese, beer, yeast products, and other foods high in tyramine. (**Ref. 1,** p. 119; **Ref. 4,** p. 417; **Ref. 10,** p. 1379; **Ref. 12,** pp. 126–127)

415. D. Chlorpromazine is effective in treating each of these conditions, including nausea and vomiting induced by drugs and by certain disease states, but it does not appear to control motion sickness. (**Ref. 4,** pp. 404, 927; **Ref. 10,** pp. 1412, 1416)

416. D. Phenothiazine antipsychotics include chlorpromazine, fluphenazine, perphenazine, prochlorperazine, thioridazine, and others. Prochlorperazine is used primarily for its antiemetic effects. Patient response to phenothiazines is variable, and those who do not respond to one may be treated successfully with another. (**Ref. 4,** p. 395; **Ref. 10,** p. 1412)

417. A. Although phenothiazines do influence neuroendocrine activity through depression of the hypothalamus, chlorpromazine has been shown to stimulate, rather than depress, milk formation, partly as a result of inhibition of prolactin-release-inhibiting hormone by the hypothalamus. (**Ref. 4,** pp. 392–393; **Ref. 10,** p. 1414)

418. B. Phenothiazines have many effects on the endocrine system. Chlorpromazine in particular seems to impair glucose tolerance and insulin release to a degree that is clinically significant in some patients. (**Ref. 4,** pp. 392–393)

419. C. The risk of seizures seems to be higher (3.5% vs. 1%) with clozapine than with other antipsychotic agents. Risk appears to be associated with dose and/or plasma levels. (**Ref. 6,** p. 876; **Ref. 10,** p. 1435)

420. B. Lithium carbonate is given to replace sodium in the body. The lithium level of around 1mEq/L in the serum is an average antipsychotic concentration. If this concentration is exceeded, tremors and mental confusion may occur. The lithium ion decreases thyroid function. Polydipsia and polyuria are frequent but reversible. Edema and weight gain occur. (**Ref. 1,** p. 407; **Ref. 4,** p. 418; **Ref. 10,** pp. 1543–1544)

421. A. Although nausea and vomiting are potential side effects of benzodiazepines, they are not used to induce emesis. They are used in the treatment of certain anxiety-related GI disorders. (**Ref. 4,** pp. 352, 346; **Ref. 6,** pp. 516–517; **Ref. 10,** p. 1488; **Ref. 12,** p. 954)

422. C. The exact mechanism of action of benzodiazepines remains unclear. The prevailing belief is that they act through the potentiation of the inhibitory neurotransmitter GABA. (**Ref. 1,** pp. 311–312; **Ref. 4,** pp. 349–350; **Ref. 6,** p. 518; **Ref. 10,** p. 1488; **Ref. 12,** pp. 338–339)

423. B. Aside from nonpharmacological interventions, benzodiazepines are the drugs of choice for the treatment of insomnia. Most commonly, patients are started on temazepam 15 to 30 mg at bedtime. (**Ref. 4,** p. 370; **Ref. 6,** pp. 517, 534; **Ref. 10,** p. 1511)

424. E. For the treatment of agitation associated with alcohol withdrawal, 50 to 100 mg of chlordiazepoxide is given intravenously. This dose may be repeated in 2 to 4 hours if needed. (**Ref. 6,** pp. 517, 524; **Ref. 10,** pp. 1495–1496; **Ref. 12,** pp. 345, 356)

425. D. IV diazepam is considered the drug of choice for acute management of status epilepticus. The initial dose in adults is 5 to 10 mg. This may be repeated every 10 to 15 minutes until a maximum of 30 mg has been given. (**Ref. 4,** pp. 455, 459; **Ref. 6,** p. 528; **Ref. 10,** p. 1498; **Ref. 12,** p. 378)

426. C. Meprobamate has been shown to precipitate seizures when used in patients with seizure disorders. (**Ref. 4,** p. 366; **Ref. 6,** p. 1840; **Ref. 10,** p. 1528)

427. A. Chloral hydrate is particularly useful in the sedation of infants, children, and the elderly. Dosage adjustments must be made, especially in the elderly for declining hepatic function. (**Ref. 6,** p. 787; **Ref. 10,** p. 1519)

428. **B.** Clonazepam is a benzodiazepine derivative classified as an anticonvulsant. It is used primarily in the prophylactic treatment of petit mal, akinetic, and myoclonic seizures. (**Ref. 4,** p. 456; **Ref. 6,** p. 525; **Ref. 10,** p. 1353; **Ref. 12,** p. 374)

429. **B.** Buspirone has similar anxiolytic activity as the benzodiazepines with the added advantage of being less sedating. The most common adverse effects of buspirone are dizziness, headache, light-headedness, and drowsiness. (**Ref. 4,** p. 428; **Ref. 6,** p. 633; **Ref. 10,** p. 1515; **Ref. 12,** pp. 342–343)

430. **D.** Flumazenil binds to benzodiazepine receptors with a higher affinity than do the benzodiazepines. Currently it is used to reverse the sedative effects in cases of benzodiazepine toxicity. (**Ref. 4,** p. 356; **Ref. 6,** p. 2842; **Ref. 10,** p. 2457; **Ref. 12,** p. 342)

431. **A.** Fluoxetine exerts most of its effects on serotonin and has little effect on other neurotransmitters. It is particularly useful in that the side effects associated with it are minimal. (**Ref. 4,** p. 406; **Ref. 6,** p. 1407; **Ref. 10,** p. 1395; **Ref. 12,** p. 453)

432. **E.** Midazolam is a benzodiazepine used for sedation during procedures such as endoscopy, cytoscopy, and bronchoscopy. It is advantageous over other agents because of its amnestic effects. (**Ref. 1,** pp. 359–360; **Ref. 4,** p. 304; **Ref. 6,** p. 1922; **Ref. 10,** p. 1504; **Ref. 12,** pp. 339, 391)

433. **C.** Phenobarbital is used in the prophylactic management of generalized tonic-clonic seizures. Its sedative effects and effects on behavior in general in children have limited its use. (**Ref. 4,** p. 945; **Ref. 6,** p. 483; **Ref. 10,** p. 1485; **Ref. 12,** p. 341)

434. **B.** All of these effects have been observed in individuals following the use of LSD, but the earliest and most persistent effect is mydriasis, which occurs even with small doses. (**Ref. 1,** p. 444; **Ref. 4,** pp. 554, 556; **Ref. 12,** p. 486)

435. **D.** Periodic measurements of lithium blood levels are required throughout treatment. This is especially important if new drugs are

introduced into the patient's regimen or if there are changes in the health status of the patient. (**Ref. 1,** pp. 406–407; **Ref. 6,** p. 1772; **Ref. 10,** p. 1544; **Ref. 12,** p. 444)

436. A. Tremor is one of the most common side effects of the use of lithium. It has been treated with propranolol with some success. (**Ref. 1,** p. 407; **Ref. 4,** pp. 420–421; **Ref. 6,** p. 1773; **Ref. 10,** pp. 1543–1544; **Ref. 12,** pp. 444–445)

437. C. Sertraline is a napthelenamine derivative antidepressant similar neither in structure nor in function to other agents. It acts primarily by inhibition of serotonin uptake but has some effect on the uptake of dopamine and norepinephrine. (**Ref. 6,** p. 2454; **Ref. 10,** p. 1406; **Ref. 12,** p. 453)

438. A. The mechanism of action of ethchlorvynol's sedative-hypnotic effects remains unknown after many years of use. It has largely been replaced by newer agents and is used only in patients refractory to other agents or in those patients with allergies to newer agents. (**Ref. 1,** p. 314; **Ref. 6,** p. 1326; **Ref. 10,** p. 1522; **Ref. 12,** p. 343)

439. E. Signs of lithium toxicity include profuse nausea and vomiting, tremor, ataxia, coma, and convulsions. It is important to warn patients of these signs, since early recognition of GI effects can enable patients to seek medical attention in a timely manner. (**Ref. 4,** p. 420; **Ref. 6,** p. 1773; **Ref. 10,** pp. 1543–1544)

440. B. Estazolam is indicated only for use in the treatment and prevention of transient insomnia. The usual dose in adults is 1 to 2 mg. (**Ref. 6,** p. 530; **Ref. 10,** pp. 1499–1500)

441. D. Flurazepam has a half life of approximately 50 to 100 hours. This extended duration in the body contributes to the hangover effect experienced by many patients. (**Ref. 4,** p. 357; **Ref. 6,** p. 530; **Ref. 10,** p. 1490; **Ref. 12,** pp. 336–337)

442. B. Patient age, drug half life, drug absorption, and underlying disorder are all important when choosing a benzodiazepine for treatment of insomnia. Other considerations are cost, concurrent medications, and other disease states. (**Ref. 4,** pp. 369–370; **Ref. 6,** p. 1490; **Ref. 12,** p. 344)

443. D. Barbiturates interact with many drugs due to their induction effects on hepatic microsomal enzymes. This can enhance the metabolism of endogenous steroids, thus leading to endocrine disturbances. (**Ref. 4,** p. 362; **Ref. 6,** pp. 475–476; **Ref. 10,** p. 1478)

444. D. Through induction of hepatic microsomal enzymes, barbiturates increase the metabolism of oral contraceptives, thus decreasing their efficacy. It is important to counsel patients concerning this effect. (**Ref. 1,** p. 318; **Ref. 6,** p. 475; **Ref. 10,** p. 1478)

445. D. Thiopental is the prototype ultra-short-acting barbiturate. Because of their short half lives, these agents are not used as sedatives, but instead are used in the induction of anesthesia. (**Ref. 1,** p. 359; **Ref. 4,** pp. 363–364; **Ref. 6,** p. 146; **Ref. 12,** pp. 390–391)

446. A. Alprazolam is available in oral dosage forms only. It is commonly used for the management of anxiety disorders and also in the management of panic disorder. (**Ref. 4,** p. 428; **Ref. 6,** p. 523)

447. E. Chlorazepate is indicated for the treatment of partial seizures in addition to its use as an anxiolytic. It has also been used in the management of agitation associated with acute ethanol withdrawal. (**Ref. 4,** p. 454; **Ref. 6,** p. 526; **Ref. 10,** p. 1496)

448. B. Amobarbital has a half life of 8 to 42 hours. (**Ref. 4,** p. 357)

449. C. The only approved indication for disulfiram is in the treatment of chronic alcoholism. When given to a patient prior to ethanol ingestion, it raises the acetaldehyde levels, contributing to a hangover effect that is meant to be a deterrent to drinking. (**Ref. 1,** pp. 326–327; **Ref. 4,** p. 378; **Ref. 6,** pp. 1203–1204; **Ref. 10,** p. 2450; **Ref. 12,** pp. 356–357)

450. B. Wernicke-Korsakoff syndrome is associated with a thiamine deficiency. It is manifested as paralysis of external eye muscles, ataxia, amnesia, and mental impairment. It is rarely seen in nonalcoholic patients. (**Ref. 1,** pp. 322–323; **Ref. 4,** p. 1533; **Ref. 12,** p. 353)

451. A. Benzodiazepines are not used in the treatment of depression. Lorazepam has been used in the treatment of nausea and vomiting associated with cancer chemotherapy. (**Ref. 1,** pp. 312–313; **Ref. 6,** p. 577; **Ref. 10,** pp. 1489–1490)

452. E. Dehydrated alcohol is injected in close proximity to nerves or basal ganglia. This effectively destroys the nerves it contacts and provides relief of neuropathic pain. Ethanol is also used in the treatment of methanol poisoning. (**Ref. 1,** p. 327; **Ref. 4,** p. 377)

453. E. Following administration, ultra-short-acting barbiturates easily cross the blood-brain barrier due to their high lipid solubility. However, their lipid solubility also allows for rapid redistribution to other tissues once in the brain. (**Ref. 1,** pp. 308–309; **Ref. 4,** p. 358; **Ref. 12,** pp. 335–336)

454. C. Recent studies have shown that ingestion of small amounts of ethanol increase the blood concentration of high density lipoproteins while lowering the concentration of low density lipoproteins. This translates to a lower incidence of coronary heart disease. (**Ref. 1,** p. 324; **Ref. 4,** p. 372; **Ref. 12,** p. 353)

455. B. Paraldehyde is a polymer of acetaldehyde. It has been used for more than a century and owing to the emergence of newer agents is seldom used today. Its most common use is in the treatment of delirium tremens. (**Ref. 4,** pp. 367–368; **Ref. 6,** pp. 2140–2141; **Ref. 10,** pp. 1531–1532)

456. C. Pentobarbital has a half-life of 15 to 48 hours. Its onset of action is 10 to 15 minutes and duration of action is 3 to 4 hours. It is used as a sedative-hypnotic and an anticonvulsant. (**Ref. 6,** p. 486; **Ref. 10,** pp. 1483–1484)

457. D. Phenobarbital has been used in the treatment of seizures associated with tetanus, meningitis, and toxic reactions to strychnine. It is also used in the prophylaxis and treatment of febrile seizures. (**Ref. 6,** p. 473; **Ref. 10,** pp. 350–351)

458. E. Oxazepam is a metabolite ot chlorazepate. It is used as a single agent in the treatment of anxiety disorders. (**Ref. 6,** p. 533; **Ref. 10,** pp. 1489, 1508)

459. A. Midazolam provides relief of anxiety prior to a procedure as well as anterograde amnesia of perioperative events. It is also used in conscious sedation, either alone or with an opiate agonist. (**Ref. 6,** pp. 1922–1923; **Ref. 10,** p. 1504; **Ref. 12,** p. 391)

460. D. Benzodiazepines have been proven to shorten the actual time spent in REM sleep while increasing the number of cycles of REM sleep in a given time period. It is still unclear how this affects overall sleep patterns. (**Ref. 1,** p. 312; **Ref. 4,** p. 349; **Ref. 12,** p. 340)

461. E. Diazepam is used as an adjunct to analgesics but not as an analgesic itself. Its benefit in analgesia is in that its anxiolytic effects may potentiate the analgesic effects of other agents. (**Ref. 6,** p. 527; **Ref. 10,** pp. 1497–1498)

462. D. Although excessive chronic consumption of alcohol results in the accumulation of fat and protein in the liver, which may proceed to cirrhosis, this is not part of the syndrome seen in the newborn. (**Ref. 1,** p. 324; **Ref. 3,** p. 344; **Ref. 4,** p. 373; **Ref. 12,** p. 354)

7

Autacoids, Analgesics, and Antipyretics

DIRECTIONS (Questions 463–476): Each of the questions or incomplete statements below is followed by five suggested answers or completions. Select the **one** that is best in each case.

463. Which of the following statements concerning angiotensin is false?
    A. Causes strong contractions of precapillary arterioles of skin, kidneys, and splanchnic area
    B. Increases the force of cardiac contractions, most likely by facilitating calcium entry, as calcium channel blockers prevent this positive inotropic action
    C. Increases aldosterone secretion by the adrenals
    D. Has no direct action on the brain because the blood-brain barrier prevents its entry
    E. Increases ADH secretion

464. When migraine is treated with ergotamine, all of the following are true EXCEPT
    A. vasoconstriction develops
    B. the carotid artery pulsation is reduced
    C. treatment is most effective if given after the attack begins
    D. the vasomotor center is depressed
    E. headache relief with ergotamine is diagnostic of migraine arterioles

465. Antihistamines (H_1) have varied clinical uses including
  A. decreased gastric secretion in peptic ulcer
  B. treatment of severe bronchial asthma episodes
  C. increased blood flow to extremities in peripheral vascular disease
  D. treatment of cardiac arrhythmias
  E. prophylaxis and treatment of motion sickness induced by air, sea, or land travel

466. Antihistamines (H_1 antagonists) are useful in treating certain allergic disorders and the mechanism is most likely the result of
  A. inhibition of histamine release
  B. depletion of histamine stores
  C. metabolic inactivation of histamine
  D. inhibition of histamine action at histamine receptors
  E. chelation of histamine

467. Concerning serotonin antagonists, all of the following statements are true EXCEPT
  A. antagonism may involve several different mechanisms
  B. antagonism by cyproheptadine is an example of surmountable competitive type
  C. methysergide is of greatest benefit during migraine attacks
  D. antagonism of the effects of serotonin can be demonstrated with chlorpromazine and phenoxybenzamine
  E. antagonism can be achieved with numerous lysergic acid derivatives, many of which are naturally occurring ergot alkaloids

468. Histamine shock is associated with all of the following EXCEPT
  A. reduced venous return to the heart
  B. a decreased effective blood volume
  C. increased capillary permeability and edema
  D. engorged large blood vessels
  E. hemoconcentration

469. The H_2-receptor antagonists selectively block gastric acid secretion EXCEPT
  A. when stimulated by histamine
  B. when stimulated by gastrin
  C. from vagus nerve stimulation with electrical stimuli
  D. when caused by atropine
  E. nocturnal gastric secretions

470. Which of the statements concerning cyproheptadine is false?
   A. Side effects include dry mouth and drowsiness
   B. It reduces smooth muscle responses from carcinoid tumors
   C. It is effective in relieving the dumping syndrome that occurs after gastrectomy
   D. It is classified as an α-adrenergic antagonist
   E. Structurally it resembles the phenothiazine antihistamines

471. All of the following statements are true of histamine EXCEPT
   A. it is stored in mast cells and basophils
   B. mast cells quickly restore the depletion of histámine
   C. it activates the phosphatidyl-inositol cycle
   D. it is a neurotransmitter
   E. it causes the "triple response"

472. Kinins are more potent than histamine on the vascular system and when injected intravenously produce all of the following effects EXCEPT
   A. brief fall in mean arterial blood pressure
   B. rapid fall in mean arterial blood pressure
   C. vasodilatation of blood vessels of the liver, kidney, heart, and skeletal muscle
   D. rapid dilation of the veins
   E. throbbing, burning pain

473. Captopril is an inhibitor of converting enzyme in the renin-angiotensin system. Which of the following statements is NOT true regarding captopril?
   A. Blocks the conversion of angiotensin I to angiotensin II
   B. Effective orally
   C. Used in the therapy of congestive heart failure
   D. Used in the treatment of hypertension
   E. Stimulates degradation of bradykinin

474. Renin secretion is inhibited by all of the following EXCEPT
   A. increased sodium ion
   B. propranolol
   C. decreased blood volume
   D. increased blood pressure
   E. angiotensin II

475. Angiotensin I acted upon by the converting enzyme, a dipeptidyl carboxypeptidase, yields angiotensin II. All of the following statements regarding angiotensin II are true EXCEPT

    A. increases the systolic and diastolic blood pressure
    B. acts on the central nervous system to induce drinking
    C. causes renal blood-vessel dilatation
    D. stimulates aldosterone biosynthesis and release
    E. increases ACTH secretion

476. Intravenously injected histamine in man exerts a variety of pharmacodynamic effects including those listed below EXCEPT

    A. abrupt fall in the arterial blood pressure
    B. an increase in heart rate
    C. bronchoconstriction
    D. increased gastric secretion
    E. the "triple response"

DIRECTIONS (Questions 477–479): The group of questions below consists of five lettered headings followed by a list of numbered phrases. For each numbered phrase, select the **one** lettered heading that is most closely associated with it. Each lettered heading may be selected once, more than once, or not at all.

    A. Cimetidine
    B. Sumatriptan
    C. Bradykinin
    D. Cyproheptadine
    E. Diphenylhydantoin

477. Used in the treatment of migraine headache

478. Antihistamine with potent antiserotonin activity

479. Effective in the treatment of the Zollinger-Ellison syndrome

DIRECTIONS (Questions 480–485): Each of the questions or incomplete statements below is followed by five suggested answers or completions. Select the **one** that is best in each case.

480. Which of the following effects is caused by prostaglandin I_2?
A. Bronchodilation
B. Inhibition of renin secretion
C. Relaxation of gastrointestinal circular muscle
D. Stimulation of gastric acid and pepsin secretion
E. Contraction of the pregnant uterus

481. Concerning the effects of eicosanoids on formed elements of blood, which of the following statements is NOT true?
A. Prostaglandin I_2 inhibits platelet aggregation
B. Prostacyclin inhibits aggregation
C. Thromboxane A_2 is a potent stimulator of platelet aggregation
D. Acetylsalicylic acid promotes platelet aggregation in women
E. LTB_4 is a chemotactic agent

482. Concerning captopril, which of the following statements is incorrect?
A. Serious toxicity may include bone marrow depression
B. Administered orally, hypotension occurs and continues for slightly more than 4 hours
C. It is indicated for acute renal stenosis
D. Minor toxicity includes loss of taste
E. NSAIDs may impair the hypotensive action

483. All of the following about the "triple response" produced by histamine are true EXCEPT
A. An early central red spot
B. A red flare of 1 or 2 cm in size appearing later
C. A white wheal replacing the original red spot
D. A long-lasting central red spot that gradually enlarges
E. It occurs after an intradermal injection

484. Vasoactive polypeptides include all of the following EXCEPT
A. vasopressin
B. substance P
C. bradykinin
D. serotonin
E. endothelin

485. Untoward effects of H_2-receptor antagonists include all of the following EXCEPT

    A. constipation
    B. headache and dizziness
    C. skin rashes
    D. a high incidence of blood dyscrasias
    E. loss of libido

DIRECTIONS (Questions 486–491): The group of questions below consists of five lettered headings followed by a list of numbered phrases or statements. For each numbered phrase or statement, select the **one** lettered heading that is most closely associated with it. Each lettered heading may be selected once, more than once, or not at all.

Questions 486–488:

    A. Acetylsalicylic acid
    B. Acetylcysteine
    C. Colchicine
    D. Acetaminophen
    E. Sulfinpyrazone

486. Effective in the treatment of gout by inhibition of the movement of leukocytes into the inflamed joint

487. Inhibits the synthesis of prostaglandins

488. An antipyretic aniline derivative with weak anti-inflammatory activity

Questions 489–491:

    A. Mefenamic acid
    B. Diflunisal
    C. Naproxen
    D. Ibuprofen
    E. Tolmetin sodium

489. Used clinically for the relief of mild to moderate pain when therapy will not exceed 1 week

490. A nonsteroidal anti-inflammatory drug with a half-life of 14 hours

491. A salicylic acid derivative three to four times more potent than aspirin as an analgesic in treatment of osteoarthritis and musculoskeletal strains or pains

---

DIRECTIONS (Questions 492–497): Each of the questions or incomplete statements below is followed by five suggested answers or completions. Select the **one** that is best in each case.

---

492. During mild chronic salicylate toxicity, the patient can be expected to experience all of the following EXCEPT
A. nausea and possibly vomiting
B. vertigo
C. tinnitus
D. metabolic acidosis
E. reduced auditory acuity

493. In severe aspirin toxicity in children, subsequent to the stage of compensated respiratory alkalosis, there develops
A. impaired hemostasis
B. compensated acidosis
C. metabolic acidosis
D. uncompensated alkalosis
E. gastric intolerance

494. The primary analgesic action of salicylates is the result of
A. a peripheral effect
B. a cortical effect
C. a hypothalamic effect
D. a change in acid-base balance
E. a lowering of the irritability of the reticular pathways

495. Which of the following statements about aspirin is NOT true?
A. Aspirin inhibits platelet aggregation
B. Aspirin is uricosuric
C. At usual dosage the main adverse effect is gastric irritation
D. Enteric coating is not sufficient to prevent gastritis
E. Heavy NSAID use is associated with gastric and duodenal ulcers

496. Which of the following is used for its keratolytic action?
  A. Aspirin
  B. Salicylic acid
  C. Methyl salicylate
  D. Difusinal
  E. Salsalate

497. Epinephrine is the drug of choice for treating this adverse effect of aspirin
  A. inhibition of hemostasis
  B. respiratory alkalosis
  C. hypersensitivity
  D. acute rheumatic fever
  E. rheumatoid arthritis

Autacoids, Analgesics, and Antipyretics

Answers and Discussion

463. **D.** Angiotensin does enter the brain, but in only a few areas. It can cause dipsosis and elevated sympathetic outflow from the brain. (**Ref. 1,** p. 252; **Ref. 4,** pp. 754–755; **Ref. 12,** p. 278)

464. **C.** Ergotamine is most effective if administered during the prodrome of an attack. Its effectiveness decreases if not administered early. It should not be administered repeatedly. (**Ref. 1,** p. 245; **Ref. 4,** pp. 940, 942–944; **Ref. 12,** p. 270)

465. **E.** Cyclizine, promethazine, and meclizine (H_1 antagonists) are widely used in the prophylaxis of motion sickness. This action may relate to their anticholinergic and/or hypnotic effects. The best clinical results with H_1 antagonists are obtained in seasonal rhinitis, in which sneezing rhinorrhea and itching of the eyes, nose, and throat are relieved. (**Ref. 1,** pp. 235–236; **Ref. 4,** pp. 587–588; **Ref. 12,** p. 258)

466. **D.** The H_1 antagonists are the competitive type. They have negligible effect on H_2 receptors. (**Ref. 1,** p. 233; **Ref. 2,** p. 997; **Ref. 4,** p. 582; **Ref. 6,** p. 623; **Ref. 12,** p. 258)

467. **C.** Methysergide, a potent serotonin antagonist, is useful only for the prevention and not for the treatment of migraine headaches. (**Ref. 1,** p. 246; **Ref. 4,** p. 595; **Ref. 12,** p. 270)

468. **D.** Large blood vessels in histamine shock are collapsed and virtually emptied of blood, whereas the fine vessels are engorged. (**Ref. 4,** p. 580)

469. **D.** These tests are all used for the classification of the H_2 receptor antagonists. (**Ref. 1,** p. 238; **Ref. 4,** pp. 899–900; **Ref. 12,** pp. 259–260)

470. **D.** Cyproheptadine is classified as a serotonin-receptor antagonist. (**Ref. 1,** p. 242; **Ref. 4,** p. 596; **Ref. 12,** p. 265)

471. **B.** Histamine is present in many cells of the body and the mast cells require approximately 2 weeks to restore their histamine content if it is depleted. (**Ref. 1,** pp. 230, 232; **Ref. 4,** p. 576; **Ref. 12,** p. 252)

472. **D.** The kinins have a marked relaxing effect on the various arterial blood vessels of the bodily organs; however, the veins react with constriction. (**Ref. 1,** p. 256; **Ref. 4,** pp. 590–591; **Ref. 12,** pp. 281–282)

473. **E.** Captopril and related converting-enzyme inhibitors are easy to administer and are used to treat various cardiovascular diseases. These compounds inhibit the degradation of body kinin. (**Ref. 1,** p. 253; **Ref. 4,** p. 757; **Ref. 12,** p. 279)

474. **D.** Renin secretion is inhibited by a number of peptides and changes in serum sodium also alter secretion. Angiotensin I is nearly inactive on the biologic systems studied. Increased blood volume inhibits renin release. (**Ref. 1,** p. 253; **Ref. 4,** p. 750; **Ref. 12,** pp. 277, 279)

475. **C.** While angiotensin I is nearly inactive, angiotensin II, which is a smaller peptide, is very active when injected into a local area such as the cerebral ventricle, where it induces polydipsia. Renal blood vessels are constricted. (**Ref. 1,** pp. 251–252; **Ref. 4,** p. 753; **Ref. 12,** p. 278)

476. **E.** The "triple response" is the result of intradermal injection of histamine. (**Ref. 1,** pp. 230–232; **Ref. 4,** p. 580; **Ref. 12,** p. 254)

477. **B.** Sumatriptan is a partially-selective inhibitor of serotonin receptors used for migraine headache treatment. (**Ref. 1,** p. 241; **Ref. 12,** p. 265)

478. **D.** Cyproheptadine is a potent inhibitor of histamine and serotonin, with some weak anticholinergic activity. It may be effective in postgastrectomy dumping syndrome. (**Ref. 1,** p. 242; **Ref. 4,** p. 596; **Ref. 12,** p. 265)

479. **A.** Cimetidine causes a significant reduction in diurnal gastric acid secretion, reduces severity of peptic ulcers, and has been found to be effective in the treatment of the Zollinger-Ellison syndrome, which is due to slow-growing localized gastrin-secreting tumors in the pancreas and duodenum. (**Ref. 1,** p. 239; **Ref. 4,** p. 902; **Ref. 12,** pp. 261–262)

480. **A.** PGI_2 inhibits gastric acid secretion, promotes secretion of renin, contracts gastrointestinal circular muscle, and causes relaxation in uterus muscle from pregnant women. It causes bronchodilation. (**Ref. 1,** p. 270; **Ref. 4,** pp. 606–607; **Ref. 12,** p. 297)

481. **D.** Aspirin inhibits platelet aggregation by inhibiting the generation of thromboxane A_2. Prostacyclin and PGI_2 are the same compound. (**Ref. 1,** p. 270; **Ref. 2,** p. 479; **Ref. 4,** pp. 606–607; **Ref. 12,** p. 297)

482. **C.** Captopril is contraindicated in patients with acute renal failure, especially with bilateral or unilateral renal artery stenosis. (**Ref. 1,** p. 157; **Ref. 4,** p. 759; **Ref. 12,** p. 165)

483. **D.** The triple response results from intradermal injection of histamine and consists of (1) a central red spot (2) surrounded by a red flare of 1 to 2 cm, and (3) a white wheal replacing the original small red spot after about 2 minutes, due to edema. (**Ref. 1,** p. 232; **Ref. 4,** p. 580; **Ref. 12,** p. 254)

484. **D.** Serotonin, or 5-hydroxytryptamine, is not a peptide. (**Ref. 1,** pp. 255–259; **Ref. 4,** pp. 588, 592, 733; **Ref. 12,** pp. 262–263)

485. D. The H_2-receptor antagonists are well-tolerated, with only a small percentage of patients complaining of headache, dizziness, and sometimes constipation or vomiting. Long-term therapy is associated with loss of libido, impotence, and gynecomastia. Cimetidine is associated with a few cases of blood dyscrasias, making the condition rare considering the high-volume usage of this drug. (**Ref. 1,** p. 239; **Ref. 4,** p. 900; **Ref. 12,** p. 262)

486. C. Colchicine also interferes with the deposition of urates in the joint by reducing the lactic acid content within the joint. (**Ref. 1,** p. 507; **Ref. 2,** p. 504; **Ref. 4,** pp. 674–675; **Ref. 12,** p. 553)

487. A. Aspirin, indomethacin, ibuprofen, and naproxen inhibit the synthesis of prostaglandins, which appears to be the mechanism responsible for their anti-inflammatory activity. (**Ref. 1,** p. 493; **Ref. 2,** p. 432; **Ref. 4,** pp. 639–641, 657; **Ref. 12,** pp. 538–540)

488. D. Acetaminophen is more effective in treating minor pain and as an antipyretic. It has weak anti-inflammatory activity and is a weak inhibitor of cyclooxygenase (prostaglandin synthase). (**Ref. 1,** pp. 493, 506; **Ref. 2,** p. 436; **Ref. 4,** pp. 656–657; **Ref. 12,** pp. 551–552)

489. A. Although mefenamic acid has anti-inflammatory effects, its propensity for causing serious side effects limits its potential usefulness to short-term therapy. (**Ref. 1,** p. 499; **Ref. 2,** p. 437; **Ref. 4,** p. 662; **Ref. 12,** p. 545)

490. C. Naproxen has pharmacological activity similar to that of ibuprofen. It has a long (14 hour) half life and is now available over the counter. (**Ref. 1,** p. 498; **Ref. 2,** p. 492; **Ref. 4,** p. 466; **Ref. 12,** p. 544)

491. B. Diflunisal possesses significant anti-inflammatory but little antipyretic activity. It does not produce auditory side effects and appears to be less irritating than aspirin to gastrointestinal mucosa. (**Ref. 1,** p. 499; **Ref. 2,** p. 433; **Ref. 4,** p. 653; **Ref. 12,** p. 542)

492. D. In addition to nausea, vertigo, tinnitus, and reduced hearing, headache and lassitude will most likely be present. Metabolic acidosis occurs with severe toxicity. (**Ref. 1,** p. 446; **Ref. 2,** p. 435; **Ref. 4,** p. 651; **Ref. 12,** pp. 541–542)

493. B. Toxic quantities of aspirin initially increase respiration, thereby reducing plasma CO_2, which results in renal excretion of sodium and potassium. Later, aspirin depresses respiration, allowing CO_2 to increase. The body does not contain sufficient sodium to prevent the development of respiratory acidosis. Gastric intolerance and impaired hemostasis are signs associated with clinically-effective levels of salicylate. (**Ref. 1,** pp. 495–496; **Ref. 2,** p. 435; **Ref. 4,** p. 651; **Ref. 12,** pp. 541–542)

494. A. Salicylates inhibit the synthesis of prostaglandins in many areas including the peripheral tissues, thus interfering with sensitization of peripheral nerve endings to pain; they also reduce the irritability of the hypothalamus. However, most sources consider the primary pain relief to occur through peripheral action. (**Ref. 1,** p. 493; **Ref. 2,** p. 435; **Ref. 4,** p. 651; **Ref. 12,** pp. 538, 540)

495. D. Most buffered aspirin still causes gastric irritation; however, enteric coating may provide effective plasma levels without irritating the stomach. (**Ref. 1,** p. 495; **Ref. 4,** pp. 642, 649; **Ref. 12,** p. 541)

496. B. All of these agents are salicylates; however, only salicylic acid is used for its keratolytic effect. It is employed in locally applied preparations for treatment of warts, corns, and fungal infections. (**Ref. 1,** p. 883; **Ref. 2,** pp. 434–435; **Ref. 4,** pp. 445, 449; **Ref. 12,** pp. 943–944)

497. C. The acute anaphylactic reaction observed in some individuals seems to be most closely related to the acetylated salicylate. The first two choices are not managed with epinephrine and the last two choices are not adverse effects but therapeutic uses. (**Ref. 1,** p. 496; **Ref. 2,** pp. 435, 488; **Ref. 4,** p. 652; **Ref. 12,** pp. 541–542)

8

Gastrointestinal Drugs

DIRECTIONS (Questions 498-507): Each group of questions below consists of lettered headings followed by a list of numbered phrases or statements. For each numbered phrase or statement, select the **one** lettered heading that is most closely associated with it. Each lettered heading may be selected only once.

A. Misoprostol
B. Omeprazole
C. Ranitidine
D. Pirenzepine
E. Sucralfate

498. An H_2-receptor antagonist

499. A prodrug that inhibits the proton pump

500. Binds to ulcerated tissue and acts as a protective barrier

501. Should not be used in patients who are pregnant and should be used with caution in women of childbearing age

502. An antimuscarinic agent useful as an adjunct to H_2-receptor antagonists

    A. Metoclopramide
    B. Diphenoxylate
    C. Ursodiol
    D. Prochlorperazine
    E. Pancrease

503. An opioid derivative used as an antidiarrheal

504. A phenothiazine used in the treatment of nausea and vomiting

505. A dopaminergic antagonist that accelerates gastric emptying

506. Decreases stool fat and nitrogen content

507. Reduces hepatic secretion of cholesterol into the bile

DIRECTIONS (Questions 508–511): Each of the incomplete statements below is followed by five suggested completions. Select the **one** that is best in each case.

---

508. All of the following statements are true concerning antiemetics EXCEPT
    A. antiemetic medications in the blood are able to cross the blood-brain barrier (BBB) and affect the chemoreceptor trigger zone because the BBB is poorly developed in this area
    B. H_1 blockers (antihistamines) are particularly useful in treating the nausea and vomiting associated with chemotherapy
    C. the mechanism of action of ondansetron and granisetron involves blockade of serotonin receptors
    D. marihuana derivatives, such as tetrahydrocannabinol, are effective antiemetics used for refractory nausea and vomiting
    E. although the primary activity of metoclopramide is to decrease intestinal transit time, it also has some antiemetic activity

509. All of the following statements concerning drugs used in the treatment of inflammatory bowel disease are true EXCEPT
    A. sulfasalazine is a pro-drug used for its anti-inflammatory effects
    B. it is necessary to supplement folic acid when taking sulfasalazine because of inhibition of folate absorption

C. cytotoxic drugs such as mercaptopurine have been used in the treatment of inflammatory bowel disease (IBD)

D. topical application of 5-aminosalicylic acid through the use of an enema is an effective prophylactic against recurrence in patients who have achieved remission

E. H_2 antagonists are useful in treating IBD

510. All of the following statements concerning antacids are true EXCEPT

A. sodium bicarbonate is very effective in neutralizing stomach acid but its use is not recommended because of the potential for systemic alkalosis and fluid retention

B. antacids only neutralize stomach acid and have no effect on the secretion of pepsin

C. a common side-effect of magnesium-based antacids is diarrhea, while aluminum-based antacids tend to cause constipation

D. milk alkali syndrome is associated with the administration of sodium bicarbonate- and calcium carbonate-containing antacids along with milk or cream

E. magnesium-based antacids, rather than aluminum-based antacids, are preferred for the treatment of patients with renal dysfunction

511. All of the following statements are true concerning laxatives EXCEPT

A. bulk-forming laxatives stimulate peristaltic action by increasing the mass in the intestine

B. the osmotic laxative, sorbitol, is also used to decrease ammonia concentrations in the blood in patients with hepatic encephalopathy

C. phenolphthalein, cascara, and senna are stimulant/irritant laxatives

D. mineral oil is not recommended for use as a laxative because it interferes with the absorption of fat-soluble vitamins

E. docusates have limited use as laxatives and are used primarily as stool softeners

Gastrointestinal Drugs

Answers and Discussion

498. C. Ranitidine acts to inhibit the secretion of gastric acid controlled by histamine release. These agents competitively bind with the histamine receptors and thus reduce the basal, nocturnal, and food-stimulated release of acid. (**Ref. 1,** p. 890; **Ref. 4,** p. 899; **Ref. 10,** p. 1945; **Ref. 12,** p. 951)

499. B. Omeprazole inhibits the second locus of control for gastric acid secretion, the proton pump. At a pH below 5, an active metabolite inactivates H^+K^+-ATPase by binding to it and thus preventing the secretion of gastric acid. (**Ref. 1,** p. 891; **Ref. 4,** p. 903; **Ref. 10,** p. 1942; **Ref. 12,** p. 952)

500. E. Sucralfate enhances ulcer healing by binding to proteins at the ulcer site and providing a protective coating against pepsin, gastric acid, and bile salts. (**Ref. 1,** p. 891; **Ref. 4,** p. 910; **Ref. 10,** p. 1950; **Ref. 12,** p. 952)

501. A. Prostaglandins E_2 and I_2 are the primary prostaglandins secreted by gastric mucosa. These substances act to increase the secretion of bicarbonate and mucus. Administration of prostaglandin analogues, such as misoprostol, provides protection for the gastric mucosa from the inhibition of prostaglandin synthesis caused by aspirin-like drugs. Misoprostol exhibits abortifacient activity and therefore should be used with caution in pregnant women or women of childbearing age. (Ref. 1, p. 891; Ref. 4, p. 911; Ref. 10, p. 1941; Ref. 12, p. 953)

502. D. Pirenzepine acts by blocking muscarinic (M_1) receptors, thereby inhibiting the cholinergic release of gastrin, mucus, and bicarbonate. (Ref. 1, p. 891; Ref. 4, p. 910; Ref. 10, p. 735-736; Ref. 12, p. 952)

503. B. Diphenoxylate is a derivative of meperidine that inhibits GI motility both locally and centrally. Atropine is often added in subtherapeutic doses to compounds containing diphenoxylate to prevent abuse of its opiate effects. (Ref. 1, p. 894; Ref. 4, p. 894; Ref. 10, p. 1877; Ref. 12, p. 956)

504. D. Prochlorperazine is a phenothiazine that acts as an antiemetic by blocking dopamine receptors in the medullary chemoreceptor trigger zone (CTZ). (Ref. 1, p. 892; Ref. 4, p. 927; Ref. 10, p. 1912-1913; Ref. 12, p. 954)

505. A. Metoclopramide, like prochlorperazine, blocks dopamine receptors in the CTZ to reduce nausea and vomiting. In addition, it increases gastric motility by increasing lower esophageal sphincter tone and stimulating peristalsis in the upper GI tract. (Ref. 1, p. 892; Ref. 4, p. 928; Ref. 10, p. 1931; Ref. 12, p. 953)

506. E. Pancrease contains primarily amylase, trypsin, and lipase, and is used in the treatment of conditions where pancreatic secretions are insufficient, such as pancreatitis. Administration of these compounds reduces the fat and nitrogen content in the stool. These parameters are used as monitors during treatment. (Ref. 1, p. 893; Ref. 4, p. 929; Ref. 10, p. 1902-1903; Ref. 12, pp. 954-955)

507. C. Ursodiol is a naturally-occurring bile acid that inhibits hepatic synthesis and secretion of cholesterol. In addition, it inhibits intestinal absorption of cholesterol. Decreased cholesterol in the bile may inhibit the formation and promote the dissolution of cholesterotic gallstones. (Ref. 1, p. 895; Ref. 4, p. 930; Ref. 12, p. 956)

508. B. H_1 blockers or antihistamines are of little use in the treatment of nausea and vomiting secondary to chemotherapy. They play a more

important role in treating nausea and vomiting associated with motion sickness. (**Ref. 1,** p. 892; **Ref. 4,** p. 927; **Ref. 10,** pp. 3, 1911; **Ref. 12,** p. 954)

509. E. H_2 blockers are ineffective in the treatment of inflammatory bowel disease because they have no anti-inflammatory or immunosuppressive effects. (**Ref. 1,** p. 895; **Ref. 12,** pp. 957–958)

510. B. Pepsin becomes inactivated as the gastric pH approaches neutrality. By increasing gastric pH, antacids inactivate pepsin. In addition, aluminum-containing antacids may have further effects due to the adsorption of pepsin to aluminum hydroxide molecules. (**Ref. 1,** pp. 888-889; **Ref. 4,** p. 905; **Ref. 10,** p. 1871; **Ref. 12,** pp. 949–950)

511. B. Lactulose, not sorbitol, is used to decrease ammonia concentrations in the blood. Metabolism of lactulose acidifies the colon, thus converting ammonia (NH_3) to ammonium (NH_4^+). The charged molecule cannot be absorbed, and is excreted in the stool. In addition, this "ion trapping" causes ammonia in the blood to diffuse into the colon, where it is excreted as well. (**Ref. 1,** p. 896; **Ref. 4,** p. 910; **Ref. 10,** pp. 1649–1650; **Ref. 12,** p. 958)

9

Chemotherapy

ANTIBIOTICS

512. All of the following statements are true concerning sulfonamides
EXCEPT
  A. antimicrobial activity is dependent upon the inhibition of the
     bacterial cell's ability to synthesize folate
  B. patients who are taking these drugs should be advised to keep
     well hydrated in order to prevent crystallization of the drug in
     the urine
  C. sulfonamides are used in combination with phenazopyridine
     for an additive antibacterial effect
  D. sulfacetamide is often used topically for the management of
     ophthalmic infections
  E. a major concern with these agents is the relatively high inci-
     dence of allergic reactions due to the sulfur content

513. Which of the following conditions is not susceptible to treatment
with trimethoprim-sulfamethoxazole?
  A. An uncomplicated gram-negative urinary tract infection
  B. Salmonella gastroenteritis
  C. Respiratory infections caused by *Haemophilus influenzae*
  D. *Pneumocystis carinii* pneumonia
  E. Tuberculosis

DIRECTIONS (Questions 514–518): The group of questions below consists of five lettered headings followed by a list of numbered phrases or statements. For each numbered phrase or statement, select the **one** lettered heading that is most closely associated with it. Each heading may be used only once.

    A. Gentamycin
    B. Chloramphenicol
    C. Ciprofloxacin
    D. Fluconazole
    E. Nitrofurantoin

514. A quinolone antibiotic that has activity against most gram-negative organisms

515. This antibiotic is used solely in the treatment of urinary tract infections because it is excreted too quickly to achieve adequate blood concentrations

516. An antifungal agent used to treat esophageal candidiasis in immunocompromised patients

517. Blood concentrations of this agent are closely monitored to prevent toxicity

518. This drug is rarely used in newborns because of their immature metabolic systems

DIRECTIONS (Questions 519–522): Each of the questions or incomplete statements below is followed by five suggested answers or completions. Select the **one** that is best in each case.

519. Which of the following drugs is not used in the treatment of tuberculosis?
    A. Isoniazid
    B. Rifampin
    C. Pyrazinamide
    D. Spectinomycin
    E. Ethambutol

520. All of the following statements are true concerning the penicillins EXCEPT
   A. this class of antibacterial acts by damaging the cell walls of bacteria
   B. oxacillin is not resistant to penicillinase
   C. piperacillin and ticarcillin have activity against Pseudomonas species
   D. use of any penicillin is contraindicated in a patient who has had an allergic reaction to any one penicillin
   E. the addition of clavulanic acid to amoxicillin preparations protects the drug from penicillinase

521. Which of the following antibiotics is not active against *Klebsiella pneumoniae*?
   A. Clindamycin
   B. Imipenem
   C. Ampicillin/sulbactam
   D. Ceftazidime
   E. Ciprofloxacin

522. Tetracyclines are useful in treating all of the following EXCEPT
   A. Rocky Mountain spotted fever
   B. mycoplasma pneumonia
   C. chlamydia
   D. acne
   E. staphylococcal infections

DIRECTIONS (Questions 523–527): The group of questions below consists of five lettered headings followed by a list of numbered potential side effects of drugs. For each numbered side effect, select the **one** lettered heading that is most closely associated with it. Each heading may only be used once.

   A. Cefoperazone
   B. Tetracycline
   C. Vancomycin
   D. Amikacin
   E. Chloramphenicol

523. Discoloration of teeth in children

524. Nephrotoxicity

525. Hypoprothrombinemia

526. Aplastic anemia

527. Red man syndrome

DIRECTIONS (Questions 528–530): Each of the incomplete statements below is followed by five suggested completions. Select the **one** that is best in each case.

---

528. All of the following statements are true concerning antiviral agents EXCEPT
   A. ribavirin enhances the antiviral activity of zidovudine
   B. the antiviral activity of acyclovir is essentially confined to herpes viruses
   C. intravitreal injections of ganciclovir are effective in treating cytomegalovirus retinitis
   D. administration of recombinant human interferon is an attempt to enhance the body's normal response to viral infection
   E. inhaled ribavirin is used to treat infants with respiratory syncytial virus

529. All of the following are effective in treating *Neisseria meningitidis* EXCEPT
   A. ampicillin
   B. metronidazole
   C. second generation cephalosporins
   D. ciprofloxacin
   E. erythromycin

530. Erythromycin is used to treat all of the following EXCEPT
   A. mycoplasma pneumonia
   B. legionnaires' disease
   C. methicillin-resistant *Staphylococcus aureus*
   D. chlamydial infections during pregnancy
   E. prophylaxis for bacterial endocarditis in penicillin-allergic patients

DIRECTIONS (Questions 531–535): The group of questions below consists of five lettered headings followed by a list of numbered phrases or statements. For each numbered phrase or statement, select the **one** lettered heading that is most closely associated with it. Each heading may be used only once.

    A. Clotrimazole
    B. Foscarnet
    C. Bacitracin
    D. Vidarabine
    E. Griseofulvin

531. An antibiotic most commonly used in topical preparations

532. Active against herpes, HIV, and cytomegalovirus

533. Superior to acyclovir in the treatment of herpes viruses in the CNS in neonates

534. Used to treat esophageal and vulvovaginal candidiasis

535. An antifungal used for infections of the skin, hair, and nails

DIRECTIONS (Questions 536–537): Each of the incomplete statements below is followed by five suggested completions. Select the **one** that is best in each case.

536. All of the following are second-generation cephalosporins EXCEPT
    A. cephalexin
    B. cefotetan
    C. cefonicid
    D. cefuroxime
    E. cefaclor

537. All of the following antibiotics act by inhibiting bacterial cell wall synthesis EXCEPT
   A. cephalosporins
   B. erythromycin
   C. penicillins
   D. vancomycin
   E. cycloserine

DIRECTIONS (Questions 538–542): The group of questions below consists of five lettered headings followed by a list of numbered phrases or statements. For each numbered phrase or statement, select the **one** lettered heading that is most closely associated with it. Each heading may be used only once.

   A. Amantadine
   B. Dapsone
   C. Mebendazole
   D. Nystatin
   E. Clindamycin

538. Drug of choice in the treatment of leprosy

539. A topical antifungal used for Candida infections

540. An oral antiviral with activity against influenza A

541. Used in the treatment of anaerobic infections, especially those with *Bacteroides fragilis*

542. Used in the treatment of pinworms

DIRECTIONS (Questions 543–546): Each of the incomplete statements below is followed by five suggested completions. Select the **one** that is best in each case.

543. All of the following reach therapeutic concentrations in the CNS EXCEPT
   A. ampicillin
   B. metronidazole

C. erythromycin
D. fluconazole
E. rifampin

544. All of the following drugs are used in the treatment of malaria EXCEPT
   A. quinine
   B. primaquine
   C. pyrimethamine
   D. mefloquine
   E. tetracycline

545. The drug of choice for treating asymptomatic and noninvasive amebiasis is
   A. diloxanide
   B. erythromycin
   C. emetine
   D. chloroquine
   E. a second generation cephalosporin

546. The most serious side effect of penicillin is
   A. hearing loss
   B. anaphylaxis secondary to allergy
   C. renal failure
   D. hepatitis
   E. metabolic disturbances

CANCER

DIRECTIONS (Questions 547–557): Each of the questions or incomplete statements below is followed by five suggested answers or completions. Select the one that is best in each case.

547. All of the following compounds are considered alkylating agents EXCEPT
   A. cyclophosphamide
   B. carmustine (BCNU)
   C. thiotepa
   D. fluorouracil
   E. dacarbazine

548. All of the following statements are true of cyclophosphamide EXCEPT
- **A.** it is available in both oral and intravenous dosage forms
- **B.** its use has been associated with renal tubular necrosis
- **C.** in addition to antineoplastic uses, it has been used as an immunosuppressant in transplant patients
- **D.** high doses have been associated with the syndrome of inappropriate secretion of antidiuretic hormone
- **E.** it is a cell-cycle-nonspecific agent

549. Which of the following bases is most susceptible to alkylating agents?
- **A.** Adenosine
- **B.** Cytosine
- **C.** Thymidine
- **D.** Guanine
- **E.** Uridine

550. All of the following statements are true of busulfan EXCEPT
- **A.** it is highly emetogenic
- **B.** its use has been associated with hyperuricemia
- **C.** it is available in oral dosage forms only
- **D.** high doses are used as a part of a combination regimen with cyclophosphamide in preparation for bone marrow transplantation
- **E.** it is used in the treatment of leukemias

551. Dacarbazine is used primarily to treat which of the following malignancies?
- **A.** Lung cancer
- **B.** Ovarian cancer
- **C.** Testicular cancer
- **D.** Melanoma
- **E.** Leukemias

552. All of the following antineoplastic agents are considered vesicants EXCEPT
- **A.** daunorubicin
- **B.** vincristine
- **C.** methotrexate
- **D.** idarubicin
- **E.** doxorubicin

553. All of the following statements concerning carmustine (BCNU) are true EXCEPT
  A. because of its rapid onset of action, the nadir of leukocyte and platelet counts can be expected to occur 7 to 10 days following treatment
  B. both oral and intravenous dosage forms are available
  C. carmustine is used to treat melanoma
  D. its use has been associated with pulmonary fibrosis
  E. it readily crosses the blood-brain barrier and thus is used to treat brain tumors and meningeal leukemia

554. Which of the following antimetabolites is NOT commonly used in the treatment of leukemias?
  A. Thioguanine
  B. Cytarabine
  C. Methotrexate
  D. Mercaptopurine
  E. Floxuridine

555. All of the following statements are true concerning cytarabine EXCEPT
  A. it is the most effective agent for induction of remission in acute myelocytic leukemia
  B. once in the body, it must be activated by enzymes to produce cytotoxic activity
  C. it is given intrathecally in the treatment of meningeal leukemias
  D. it is a cell-cycle-nonspecific agent
  E. it is highly emetogenic

556. Which of the following antimetabolites is only available in an oral dosage form?
  A. Mercaptopurine
  B. Bleomycin
  C. Thioguanine
  D. Methotrexate
  E. Cytarabine

557. All of the following statements concerning fluorouracil are true EXCEPT
    A. it is available as a cream
    B. it is used as a single agent in the treatment of breast cancer
    C. it causes alopecia
    D. it acts by inhibiting thymidylate synthesis
    E. it can enter the CSF

DIRECTIONS (Questions 558–562): The group of questions below consists of five potential toxicities followed by a list of chemotherapeutic agents. For each chemotherapeutic agent, select the **one** potential side effect that is most closely associated with it. Each toxicity may be used only once.

    A. Fever and chills
    B. Cystitis
    C. Neurologic toxicity
    D. Cardiomyopathy
    E. Hepatotoxicity

558. Vincristine

559. Doxorubicin

560. BCNU

561. Bleomycin

562. Ifosfamide

DIRECTIONS (Questions 563–581): Each of the questions or incomplete statements below is followed by five suggested answers or completions. Select the **one** that is best in each case.

563. Which of the following antineoplastics is NOT considered an antimetabolite?
    A. Fluorouracil
    B. Thioguanine
    C. Methotrexate

D. Pentostatin
E. Etoposide

564. All of the following statements are true of L-asparaginase EXCEPT
   A. it is used to treat acute lymphocytic leukemia
   B. it is severely emetogenic and causes life-threatening bone marrow depression
   C. it can cause severe toxicity by limiting the production of clotting factors
   D. hypersensitivity is relatively common
   E. it is an enzyme that depletes tumor cells of the amino acid asparagine

565. Vincristine is used primarily in the treatment of which of the following?
   A. Hodgkin's disease
   B. Lung cancer
   C. Liver cancer
   D. Melanoma
   E. Prostate cancer

566. One of the side effects of the antibiotic dactinomycin is
   A. pulmonary fibrosis
   B. renal damage
   C. radiation-recall reaction
   D. vaginal bleeding
   E. cardiomyopathy

567. All of the following statements concerning etoposide are true EXCEPT
   A. it is available in both injectable and oral dosage forms
   B. its dose-limiting toxicity is mucositis
   C. it is used primarily, but not exclusively, in the treatment of testicular and lung cancers
   D. mild peripheral neuropathy is a potential side effect
   E. the dose should be modified according to the patient's creatinine clearance

568. Mitoxantrone is used in the treatment of which of the following cancers?
- **A.** Leukemia
- **B.** Prostate
- **C.** Osteosarcoma
- **D.** Lung
- **E.** Renal

569. All of the following statements are true concerning tamoxifen EXCEPT
- **A.** it is more effective in postmenopausal women than in pre-menopausal women
- **B.** it is available in oral form only
- **C.** hot flashes and nausea and vomiting are the most frequently-occurring side effects
- **D.** it is used in the treatment of breast cancer
- **E.** it has been proven to be effective in treating both estrogen receptor-positive and -negative tumors

570. Leuprolide is used in the treatment of which of the following cancers?
- **A.** Pancreatic
- **B.** Non-Hodgkin's lymphoma
- **C.** Lung
- **D.** Prostate
- **E.** Liver

571. Aminoglutethimide is used in the treatment of metastatic breast cancer because of its ability to
- **A.** cross the blood-brain barrier
- **B.** inhibit the synthesis of adrenal steroids
- **C.** enhance the activity of other chemotherapeutic agents
- **D.** penetrate fatty tissue
- **E.** inactivate enzymes found in chemotherapy-resistant tumor cells

572. A cell-cycle-specific antimetabolite used in the treatment of acute myelocytic leukemia is
- **A.** lomustine
- **B.** cytarabine
- **C.** taxol
- **D.** mitomycin
- **E.** daunorubicin

573. Long-term therapy with this oral nitrogen mustard has been associated with increased incidence of leukemia.
   A. Busulfan
   B. Etoposide
   C. Methotrexate
   D. Chlorambucil
   E. Tamoxifen

574. The primary preventable toxicity associated with the administration of cisplatin is
   A. nephrotoxicity
   B. hepatocellular damage
   C. erythema at the administration site
   D. alopecia
   E. rash

575. Red-colored urine is a side effect of which of the following drugs?
   A. Cyclophosphamide
   B. Hydroxyurea
   C. Daunorubicin
   D. Methotrexate
   E. Mitomycin

576. Levamisole is used in the treatment of certain malignancies due to its
   A. low cost
   B. mild side effect profile
   C. lack of resistant tumors
   D. rapid absorption
   E. immunomodulation effects

577. Which of the following agents is used in the treatment of brain tumors?
   A. Lomustine
   B. Pentostatin
   C. Mechlorethamine
   D. L-asparaginase
   E. Vinblastine

578. Flutamide is used in the treatment of
   A. leukemias
   B. head and neck cancers
   C. lung cancer
   D. prostate cancer
   E. melanoma

579. Leucovorin is administered with methotrexate
   A. because of its additive antineoplastic effects
   B. to reverse toxic effects of methotrexate
   C. as an antiemetic
   D. to prevent renal damage
   E. to increase cellular uptake of methotrexate

580. Which of the following is a progestin used in the treatment of breast cancer?
   A. Tamoxifen
   B. Mitotane
   C. Megestrol acetate
   D. Prednisone
   E. Aminoglutethimide

581. Hydroxyurea is used in the treatment of
   A. leukemia
   B. lung cancer
   C. brain tumors
   D. pancreatic cancer
   E. breast cancer

Chemotherapy

Answers and Discussion

512. C. Phenazopyridine has no antibacterial activity. It is included in products intended for the treatment of urinary tract infections solely for its analgesic properties. (**Ref. 4,** p. 1061; **Ref. 10,** p. 2333; **Ref. 12,** pp. 716–719)

513. E. *Mycobacterium tuberculosis* is not susceptible to treatment with trimethoprim or sulfamethoxazole. Infections with this organism are treated with a combination of the following: isoniazid, rifampin, pyrazinamide, and ethambutol. (**Ref. 1,** p. 665; **Ref. 4,** pp. 1030, 1056–1057; **Ref. 10,** p. 531; **Ref. 12,** pp. 707–711)

514. C. Ciprofloxacin is used in treating gram-negative infections of the urinary tract, as well as bone and soft-tissue infections. It is active against most gram-negative bacteria, including *Enterobacteriaceae* and *Pseudomonas aeruginosa*. (**Ref. 1,** p. 686; **Ref. 4,** p. 1060; **Ref. 10,** p. 468; **Ref. 12,** p. 742)

515. E. Nitrofurantoin is rapidly and completely absorbed from the GI tract but excreted so quickly that it never reaches bactericidal concentrations in the plasma. Its half-life in the plasma is approximately 20 minutes to 1 hour. (**Ref. 1,** p. 687; **Ref. 4,** p. 1061; **Ref. 10,** pp. 520–521; **Ref. 12,** pp. 743–744)

516. D. Oral fluconazole is effective in treating both oral and esophageal candidiasis in immunocompromised patients. Its IV formulation has been used in the treatment of systemic candidal infections. (**Ref. 1,** p. 670; **Ref. 4,** p. 1172; **Ref. 10,** p. 75; **Ref. 12,** p. 726)

517. A. Gentamycin, as well as the other aminoglycosides, is associated with nephrotoxicity and ototoxicity, both of which are related to plasma concentration. Patients must be closely monitored while using these agents and their doses adjusted with changing renal function. (**Ref. 1,** p. 649; **Ref. 4,** p. 1109; **Ref. 10,** pp. 56, 61; **Ref. 12,** p. 702)

518. B. "Grey baby" syndrome is a potentially lethal condition seen in infants given chloramphenicol. Because their metabolic pathways are not fully developed, excretion of chloramphenicol is inhibited and the drug accumulates to toxic levels. (**Ref. 1,** p. 640; **Ref. 4,** pp. 1128–1129; **Ref. 10,** p. 193; **Ref. 12,** p. 694)

519. D. Spectinomycin has little activity against *Mycobacterium tuberculosis*. It is used as a single intramuscular injection in the treatment of uncomplicated gonorrhea in patients who are allergic to the drug of choice, ceftriaxone, or to penicillins. (**Ref. 1,** p. 650; **Ref. 4,** p. 1137; **Ref. 10,** p. 354; **Ref. 12,** p. 70)

520. B. All of the following penicillins are resistant to beta-lactamases: oxacillin, cloxacillin, dicloxacillin, and nafcillin. Their sole indication is in the treatment of penicillinase-producing strains of staphylococci. (**Ref. 1,** p. 630; **Ref. 4,** p. 1076; **Ref. 10,** p. 261; **Ref. 12,** p. 684)

521. A. Clindamycin and the other macrolide antibiotics have no activity against *Klebsiella pneumoniae*. Klebsiella infections of the urinary tract are treated with a second- or third-generation cephalosporin. Klebsiella pneumonia is treated with an aminoglycoside or mezlocillin or piperacillin and a third-generation cephalosporin. (**Ref. 1,** p. 697; **Ref. 4,** p. 1028; **Ref. 10,** p. 342; **Ref. 12,** p. 741)

522. E. Tetracycline is not used in the treatment of staphylococcal infections. Treatment of such infections usually involves a penicillin or, in the case of methicillin-resistant strains, vancomycin. (**Ref. 1,** pp. 642, 697; **Ref. 4,** p. 1024; **Ref. 10,** pp. 324–325; **Ref. 12,** p. 696)

523. B. Tetracyclines bind to calcium deposited in newly-forming bones and teeth. This can lead to discoloration of the teeth and deformities in the bone structure. For this reason, the use of tetracyclines should be avoided in children under six and pregnant women. (**Ref. 1,** p. 643; **Ref. 4,** p. 1122; **Ref. 10,** p. 332; **Ref. 12,** p. 697)

524. D. Amikacin, like all other aminoglycosides, can cause nephrotoxicity secondary to the accumulation of the drug in the renal tubules. This can be avoided by carefully monitoring renal function and plasma concentrations and adjusting the dose accordingly. (**Ref. 1,** pp. 647–648; **Ref. 4,** p. 1106; **Ref. 10,** p. 56; **Ref. 12,** p. 703)

525. A. Cephalosporins that contain a methylthiotetrazole group, such as cefoperazone, cefotetan, cefamandole and moxalactam can cause hypoprothrombinemia and other bleeding disorders. This is avoided by the administration of vitamin K, 10 mg twice weekly, for the duration of therapy. (**Ref. 1,** p. 635; **Ref. 4,** p. 1091; **Ref. 10,** p. 120; **Ref. 12,** p. 689)

526. E. Aplastic anemia associated with the use of chloramphenicol is somewhat rare but has occurred with long-term use. It is generally irreversible and fatal. (**Ref. 1,** p. 640; **Ref. 4,** p. 1128; **Ref. 10,** p. 193; **Ref. 12,** p. 694)

527. C. Red man syndrome is characterized by a sudden decrease in blood pressure, flushing, and/or a maculopapular or erythematous rash on the face, neck, or chest. It is believed to be caused by histamine release and has been associated with rapid infusions of vancomycin. This reaction can be prevented by infusing the drug over 1 hour or longer. (**Ref. 1,** p. 683; **Ref. 4,** p. 1139; **Ref. 10,** p. 357; **Ref. 12,** p. 738)

528. A. Concomitant administration of zidovudine and ribavirin decreases the antiviral action of zidovudine. The mechanism of this interaction is unclear, but it is postulated that ribavirin may interfere with the phosphorylation steps that convert zidovudine to its active triphosphate metabolites. (**Ref. 1,** p. 675; **Ref. 4,** p. 1183; **Ref. 10,** p. 425)

529. B. Metronidazole has no activity against *Neisseria meningitidis*. Penicillin, ampicillin, or a third-generation cephalosporin are the recommended therapy for this infection. (**Ref. 1,** p. 697; **Ref. 4,** p. 1026; **Ref. 10,** p. 539; **Ref. 12,** pp. 799–800)

530. C. Vancomycin is the drug of choice in the treatment of methicillin-resistant *Staphylococcus aureus*. (**Ref. 1,** p. 697; **Ref. 4,** pp. 1133–1134, 1140; **Ref. 10,** p. 356; **Ref. 12,** pp. 738, 740–741)

531. C. Bacitracin is used as an antibacterial agent in many over-the-counter topical creams. It is especially useful because it has a very low incidence of hypersensitivity reactions. (**Ref. 1,** p. 682; **Ref. 4,** p. 1140; **Ref. 12,** p. 739)

532. B. Foscarnet has activity against HIV, cytomegalovirus, and herpes viruses. It is especially useful in the treatment of herpes viruses resistant to both acyclovir and ganciclovir. (**Ref. 1,** p. 676; **Ref. 4,** p. 1189; **Ref. 12,** p. 734)

533. D. In the treatment of neonates with CNS involvement or visceral dissemination of the herpes virus, vidarabine is superior to acyclovir. (**Ref. 1,** p. 676; **Ref. 4,** p. 1188)

534. A. Clotrimazole is most commonly used orally in troches and in vaginal creams for the treatment of candidiasis. (**Ref. 1,** p. 669; **Ref. 4,** p. 1176; **Ref. 10,** p. 2277; **Ref. 12,** pp. 727–728)

535. E. Griseofulvin, once absorbed, has an affinity for fungal growth in skin and hair. It binds to the keratin in these areas and the new growth of tissue is free of fungus. (**Ref. 1,** p. 671; **Ref. 4,** p. 1173; **Ref. 10,** p. 83; **Ref. 12,** pp. 726–727)

536. A. Cephalexin is a first-generation cephalosporin. The second-generation cephalosporins are: cefaclor, cefamandole, cefonicid, ceforanide, cefoxitin, cefotetan, and cefuroxime. The second-generation cephalosporins have more activity against gram-negative organisms than do first-generation drugs. (**Ref. 1,** p. 634; **Ref. 4,** p. 1086; **Ref. 10,** p. 99; **Ref. 12,** pp. 687–688)

537. B. Erythromycin inhibits protein synthesis by binding to the 50S ribosomal unit in sensitive microorganisms. It exerts its effects only on actively-dividing cells. (**Ref. 1,** p. 620; **Ref. 4,** p. 1131; **Ref. 10,** pp. 194–195; **Ref. 12,** p. 740)

538. B. Dapsone is the drug of choice for the treatment of *Mycobacterium leprae* infection. Due to the emergence of resistant strains, it is now being used in combination with rifampin. (**Ref. 1**, p. 659; **Ref. 4**, pp. 1030, 1159–1160; **Ref. 10**, p. 515; **Ref. 12**, p. 713)

539. D. Nystatin is commonly used as a cream for topical infections or as a suspension for oral, esophageal, and intestinal candidiasis. (**Ref. 1**, p. 671; **Ref. 4**, p. 1179; **Ref. 10**, p. 94; **Ref. 12**, p. 727)

540. A. Amantadine has been proven to inhibit influenza A, rubella, and other viruses. However, vaccination with the influenza virus vaccine is still the preferred method of immunization. (**Ref. 1**, pp. 674–675; **Ref. 4**, p. 1192; **Ref. 10**, pp. 292–293; **Ref. 12**, pp. 730–731)

541. E. Clindamycin is the treatment of choice for *Bacteroides fragilis* infections outside the CNS. Because metronidazole reaches therapeutic concentrations in the CNS, it is preferred in CNS infections. (**Ref. 1**, p. 684; **Ref. 4**, pp. 1029, 1135–1136; **Ref. 10**, p. 343; **Ref. 12**, p. 741)

542. C. Mebendazole, 100 mg, is given once and repeated in two and four weeks in the treatment of pinworms, whipworms, roundworms, and mixed helminthic infections. (**Ref. 1**, p. 754; **Ref. 4**, p. 964; **Ref. 10**, pp. 39–40)

543. C. Erythromycin has no penetration into the CSF. Following oral or IV administration, erythromycin quickly distributes to most body tissues, excluding the brain. Drug concentrations in the tissues often are higher and persist longer than serum concentrations. (**Ref. 1**, p. 684; **Ref. 4**, p. 1132; **Ref. 10**, p. 195)

544. E. Tetracycline is not used in the treatment of malaria. Currently, chloroquine is the most commonly-used drug for the treatment and prophylaxis of this disease. (**Ref. 1**, p. 725; **Ref. 4**, p. 995; **Ref. 10**, p. 453; **Ref. 12**, pp. 782, 785)

545. A. Diloxanide is the treatment of choice for asymptomatic noninvasive amebiasis. This drug is available only by special request from the Centers for Disease Control on an investigational basis. (**Ref. 1**, p. 739; **Ref. 4**, p. 955; **Ref. 10**, p. 36; **Ref. 12**, p. 795)

212 / 9: Chemotherapy

546. B. Anaphylaxis is a life-threatening reaction involving severe hypotension and/or bronchoconstriction (incidence 1:1000). It is generally treated with epinephrine and discontinuation of and future avoidance of all penicillin derivatives. (**Ref. 1,** pp. 630–631; **Ref. 3,** pp. 649–650; **Ref. 4,** pp. 1082–1083; **Ref. 12,** pp. 684–685)

547. D. Fluorouracil is classified as an antimetabolite. It acts by competing for an enzyme required for the synthesis of thymidylate, a necessary cofactor in the synthesis of DNA. (**Ref. 1,** p. 777; **Ref. 4,** p. 1228; **Ref. 8,** pp. 400–407; **Ref. 12,** p. 834)

548. B. Cyclophosphamide has been associated with hemorrhagic cystitis in 5 to 10% of patients. It is believed to be caused by chemical irritation of the bladder by metabolites. Incidence can be reduced by adequate hydration and the administration of mesna or acetylcysteine. (**Ref. 1,** p. 774; **Ref. 4,** p. 1218; **Ref. 8,** p. 404; **Ref. 12,** p. 831)

549. D. Although all DNA bases are potentially susceptible to alkylation, the 7-nitrogen atom of guanine seems to be particularly susceptible to covalent bonding with these agents. (**Ref. 1,** p. 769; **Ref. 4,** p. 1209; **Ref. 8,** p. 400; **Ref. 12,** p. 827)

550. A. Busulfan exerts most of its cytotoxic activity solely on the bone marrow. Nausea and vomiting are side effects seen in some patients but they are less likely than with most cytotoxic agents. (**Ref. 4,** p. 1220; **Ref. 8,** p. 403; **Ref. 12,** pp. 826–829)

551. D. Dacarbazine is used predominately in the treatment of malignant melanoma. It also is used in Hodgkin's disease and various sarcomas. In the latter cases, dacarbazine is usually a part of a combination regimen with other agents such as doxorubicin, bleomycin, and vinblastine. (**Ref. 1,** p. 773; **Ref. 4,** pp. 1222–1223; **Ref. 8,** p. 1636; **Ref. 12,** p. 830)

552. C. Methotrexate is not considered a vesicant. The major toxicities associated with its use are stomatitis, alopecia, nephrotoxicity, myelosuppression, and pneumonitis. (**Ref. 1,** pp. 775–778; **Ref. 4,** pp. 1226–1227; **Ref. 8,** p. 2574; **Ref. 12,** pp. 832–833)

553. A. When using carmustine, the nadir of leukocyte and platelet counts is not reached until 4 to 6 weeks after treatment. For this reason, cyclic treatments are spaced at intervals no shorter than every 6 to 8 weeks. (Ref. 8, p. 406; Ref. 10, p. 566; Ref. 12, pp. 829–830)

554. E. Floxuridine is not used in the treatment of adult leukemias. Because almost 90% of the drug is removed in the first pass through the liver, it is predominately used in the treatment of hepatic tumors. (Ref. 4, p. 1230; Ref. 10, p. 603; Ref. 12, p. 834)

555. D. Cytarabine is cell-cycle specific for the S cycle. For this reason, it is often administered as a continuous infusion over 5 to 7 days or every 12 hours as a rapid IV injection for 5 to 7 days. (Ref. 4, pp. 1231–1232; Ref. 8, pp. 365–366; Ref. 12, pp. 834–835)

556. A. A typical dose of 6-mercaptopurine is 100mg/m^2 orally daily for maintenance of remission in some leukemias. (Ref. 4, p. 1236; Ref. 8, p. 377; Ref. 12, pp. 833–834)

557. B. Fluorouracil is always used in combination therapy when treating breast cancer. The common regimens are cyclophosphamide, doxorubicin, vincristine, and fluorouracil; or cyclophosphamide, methotrexate, and fluorouracil. (Ref. 4, p. 1230; Ref. 8, pp. 362–364; Ref. 12, p. 834)

558. C. Neurotoxicity is the dose-limiting toxicity of treatments involving vincristine. Peripheral neuropathy is often present when normal clinical doses are administered and is not severe enough to require discontinuing therapy. However, neuropathy can progress to muscle weakness of the limbs, face, and larynx, which requires discontinuation of treatment. (Ref. 4, p. 1237; Ref. 8, p. 2351; Ref. 12, p. 835)

559. D. Two types of cardiomyopathy occur following administration of doxorubicin. The first occurs in 24 to 48 hours following a dose. It is characterized by abnormal electrocardiographic studies and is usually reversible. However, this acute toxicity can in extreme cases evolve into what is known as the myocarditis-pericarditis syndrome, which can be fatal. The second type of toxicity is related to cumulative lifetime dose of the drug and results in congestive heart failure resistant to treatment with digoxin. (Ref. 4, p. 1243; Ref. 8, p. 378; Ref. 12, pp. 837–838)

560. E. Reversible hepatotoxicity has been reported in 26% of patients treated with BCNU. Signs and symptoms of this condition include increased serum transaminases, alkaline phosphatase, and bilirubin, as well as portal-system encephalopathy. **(Ref. 10,** p. 566; **Ref. 11,** p. 40)

561. A. Sixty percent of patients treated with bleomycin experience a febrile response, which may last for up to 48 hours following a single dose. The reaction is believed to be mediated by the release of histamine, and for this reason patients are often premedicated with acetaminophen and diphenhydramine. **(Ref. 4,** p. 1246; **Ref. 8,** p. 376; **Ref. 11,** p. 31; **Ref. 12,** p. 839)

562. B. Use of Ifosfamide has been associated with the development of hemorrhagic cystitis, believed to be caused by the formation of a toxic metabolite in the urine. Mesna is often administered concurrently to detoxify the metabolite. In addition, increased hydration helps to decrease the incidence of this side effect. **(Ref. 4,** p. 1218; **Ref. 8,** pp. 2350–2351; **Ref. 11,** pp. 116–117)

563. E. Etoposide is considered a plant alkaloid antineoplastic. It is a cell-cycle-specific agent that has primary activity on cells in the G_2 and late S phase. **(Ref. 4,** p. 1206; **Ref. 8,** pp. 358–371; **Ref. 9,** p. 352; **Ref. 12,** pp. 832–835)

564. B. L-asparaginase is neither emetogenic nor does it have much of an effect on the bone marrow. For this reason, it is especially useful in combination regimens, since it does not add to the bone marrow toxicity of other drugs. **(Ref. 4,** p. 1248; **Ref. 8,** pp. 387–388; **Ref. 12,** p. 842)

565. A. Vincristine is used as a component of the MOPP regimen in the treatment of Hodgkin's disease. The MOPP regimen consists of mechlorethamine, vincristine (Oncovin), procarbazine, and prednisone. **(Ref. 4,** p. 1239; **Ref. 8,** pp. 1843–1844; **Ref. 9,** p. 1718; **Ref. 11,** p. 326; **Ref. 12,** p. 835)

566. C. Administration of dactinomycin has been associated with what is known as radiation-recall reaction. This reaction manifests itself as increased inflammation, erythema, and desquamation in areas previously subjected to radiation treatments. (**Ref. 4,** p. 1240; **Ref. 8,** p. 383; **Ref. 12,** p. 838)

567. B. Leukopenia is the dose-limiting side-effect of etoposide. Leukopenia, thrombocytopenia, and anemia all occur within 7 to 14 days following treatment. (**Ref. 4,** p. 1240; **Ref. 8,** pp. 414, 327; **Ref. 9,** p. 385; **Ref. 12,** p. 836)

568. A. Mitoxantrone is used in combination regimens for the treatment of leukemias and breast cancer. (**Ref. 4,** p. 1244; **Ref. 8,** p. 1949; **Ref. 11,** p. 153; **Ref. 12,** p. 843)

569. E. Tamoxifen acts by blocking the effects of estrogens on tissues, therefore only estrogen receptor-positive tumors respond to treatment. (**Ref. 4,** p. 1256; **Ref. 8,** pp. 1308–1309, 1317; **Ref. 12,** p. 841)

570. D. Leuprolide has been used in the treatment of prostate cancer because of its effects in decreasing circulating testosterone levels through the inhibition of the secretion of LH and FSH to levels comparable with castration. (**Ref. 4,** p. 1257; **Ref. 10,** p. 645; **Ref. 12,** p. 841)

571. B. Aminoglutethimide is used in the treatment of metastatic breast cancer because of its ability to inhibit the synthesis of adrenal steroids. It has been found that breast tumor growth is related to the presence of a hormone, most likely an estrogen. Withdrawal of this hormone thus inhibits the growth of the tumor. (**Ref. 4,** p. 1254; **Ref. 8,** pp. 1318–1319; **Ref. 12,** p. 842)

572. B. Cytarabine is the most important agent used in the treatment of acute myelocytic leukemias. It is effective as a single agent with a 20 to 40% remission rate. Cytarabine is more effective when used in combination with anthracyclines, producing remission rates of greater than 50%. (**Ref. 4,** p. 1232; **Ref. 8,** p. 365; **Ref. 12,** p. 845)

573. D. Long-term administration of chlorambucil and other alkylating agents has been associated with an increased incidence of late onset leukemias. (**Ref. 4,** p. 1219; **Ref. 8,** pp. 208–209; **Ref. 11,** p. 43)

574. A. Nephrotoxicity due to cisplatin can be avoided if the patient is pretreated with hydration and diuresis. (**Ref. 4**, p. 1250; **Ref. 8**, p. 2349; **Ref. 11**, p. 47; **Ref. 12**, pp. 830–831)

575. C. Patients may notice a pink to red color in the urine for up to 48 hours following a dose of daunorubicin. (**Ref. 4**, p. 1243; **Ref. 10**, p. 594; **Ref. 11**, p. 66)

576. E. Levamisole, originally used to treat parasitic infections, has been found to increase the magnitude of T-cell–mediated immunity in humans. It has been used to treat the immunodeficiency associated with Hodgkin's disease and as an adjuvant to fluorouracil in colon cancer. (**Ref. 1**, p. 813; **Ref. 4**, p. 1230; **Ref. 8**, p. 956; **Ref. 12**, p. 810)

577. A. Because lomustine is highly lipid soluble and easily crosses the blood-brain barrier, it has been beneficial in the treatment of brain tumors. (**Ref. 1**, p. 772; **Ref. 4**, p. 1222; **Ref. 8**, p. 406; **Ref. 11**, p. 272; **Ref. 12**, pp. 829–830)

578. D. Flutamide is an antiandrogen that has been approved for the treatment of prostate cancer. The usual dose is 250 mg by mouth three times daily. Larger doses have been used experimentally with no increased benefit. (**Ref. 1**, p. 784; **Ref. 4**, p. 1207; **Ref. 8**, p. 1106; **Ref. 12**, p. 841)

579. B. Leucovorin is a folic acid derivative that is enzymatically activated to replenish the folate pool depleted by methotrexate in healthy cells. (**Ref. 1**, p. 776; **Ref. 4**, p. 1226; **Ref. 8**, p. 3604; **Ref. 12**, p. 833)

580. C. Megestrol inhibits growth and decreases the size of progestin-sensitive breast and endometrial tumors. (**Ref. 1**, pp. 782–783; **Ref. 4**, p. 1207; **Ref. 8**, p. 1318; **Ref. 12**, p. 840)

581. A. Hydroxyurea is used as a secondary agent in the treatment of chronic myelogenous leukemia. (**Ref. 1**, p. 785; **Ref. 4**, pp. 1251–1252; **Ref. 8**, p. 1972; **Ref. 12**, p. 847)

10

Toxicology

DIRECTIONS (Questions 582–587): Each of the incomplete statements below is followed by five suggested completions. Select the **one** that is best in each case.

582. All of the following statements are true concerning mercury EXCEPT
   A. mercury was once a common ingredient in pharmaceuticals, such as antibacterials and skin ointments
   B. once in the body, mercury exerts its toxicity by irreversibly binding to β-receptors
   C. symptoms of mercury poisoning include tremor, gingivitis, and personality changes
   D. elemental mercury is more toxic if inhaled than if ingested
   E. the relationship between plasma concentrations and toxicity depends on the type of exposure

583. All of the following are signs of arsenic poisoning EXCEPT
   A. severe renal damage
   B. nausea and vomiting
   C. tremor
   D. bone marrow depression
   E. cutaneous vasodilation with "milk and roses" complexion

584. All of the following statements are true concerning lead poisoning EXCEPT
   A. lead encephalopathy is more severe in children than in adults
   B. diagnosis is confirmed by measuring erythrocyte protoporphyrin
   C. chronic intoxication can result in a hypochromic microcytic anemia similar to that seen in iron deficiency
   D. chronic poisoning can be detected by x-ray studies
   E. the distribution of lead in the body closely resembles that of phosphate

585. All of the following are symptoms of chronic lead poisoning EXCEPT
   A. constipation
   B. pulmonary edema
   C. confusion/delirium
   D. nephropathy
   E. ashen skin color

586. All of the following statements are true of iron poisoning EXCEPT
   A. it is primarily seen in children
   B. if untreated, it can lead to acidosis
   C. tremor and seizures are early symptoms
   D. if death does not occur within the first six hours there may be a period of apparent recovery followed by death in 12 to 24 hours
   E. X-ray films are helpful in determining the number of tablets ingested

587. All of the following are symptoms associated with overdoses of opioids EXCEPT
   A. lethargy
   B. pinpoint pupils
   C. decreased blood pressure
   D. cool skin
   E. diarrhea

DIRECTIONS (Questions 588–593): The group of questions below consists of six antidotes followed by a list of numbered poisons. For each numbered poison, select the **one** lettered antidote that is most closely associated with it. Each heading may be used only once.

A. Pralidoxime
B. Ethanol
C. Glucagon
D. Acetylcysteine
E. Penicillamine
F. Deferoxamine

588. Acetaminophen

589. Lead

590. Methanol

591. Iron

592. β-Blockers

593. Anticholinesterases

DIRECTIONS (Questions 594–599): Each of the incomplete statements below is followed by five suggested answers or completions. Select the **one** that is best in each case.

594. All of the following statements are true concerning carbon monoxide EXCEPT
A. toxicity results from the inhibition of the oxygen-carrying capacity of hemoglobin
B. children are more susceptible to the effects of carbon monoxide because of their increased metabolic rate
C. the presence of carbon monoxide in the blood does not act as a respiratory stimulant
D. the organ most affected by carbon monoxide poisoning is the liver
E. hyperbaric conditions are used to increase excretion in the treatment of carbon monoxide poisoning

595. All of the following statements are true concerning hydrocarbons EXCEPT
   A. the primary concern in the ingestion of gasoline is the potential for aspiration
   B. in addition to its CNS depressant effects, chloroform has been identified as a potential carcinogen
   C. initial symptoms of exposure to carbon tetrachloride include CNS depression and convulsions
   D. the toxicity associated with carbon tetrachloride is believed to be associated with the reaction of free radicals with lipids and proteins
   E. halogenated hydrocarbons exert cardiotoxic effects by making the heart more sensitive to catecholamines

596. All of the following statements are true concerning benzenes EXCEPT
   A. no specific treatment exists for acute toxic exposures
   B. chronic exposure has been linked to an increased incidence of lung cancer
   C. chronic exposure results in aplastic anemia
   D. early signs of toxicity are headache and decreased appetite
   E. the major effects of short-term exposure are on the CNS

597. All of the following statements are true of methanol and isopropanol EXCEPT
   A. hemodialysis is useful in removing both agents from the blood
   B. in methanol poisoning, inebriation is a prominent symptom
   C. isopropanol produces more severe nausea and vomiting than does methanol or ethanol
   D. isopropanol is more toxic than either methanol or ethanol because it is metabolized to acetone, which acts as a CNS depressant
   E. methanol is metabolized to formic acid, which can lead to metabolic acidosis

598. All of the following are symptoms of glycol poisoning EXCEPT
   A. CNS depression
   B. metabolic acidosis
   C. acute renal failure

    D. narcosis
    E. anemia

599. Sulfur dioxide
    A. irritates mucous membranes and causes bronchoconstriction
    B. is lethal even in low concentrations
    C. poisoning is treatable if the antidote is administered within 3 hours of exposure
    D. exposure causes inflammation of neuronal membranes, leading to neuropathies
    E. is a relatively uncommon air pollutant

DIRECTIONS (Questions 600–605): Each group of questions below consists of six lettered headings followed by a list of numbered phrases or statements. For each numbered phrase or statement, select the **one** lettered heading that is most closely associated with it. Each heading may be used only once.

Questions 600–605:
    A. Paraquat
    B. Cyanide
    C. Hexachlorobenzene
    D. Malathion
    E. Strychnine
    F. DDT

600. Poisoning with this agent is characterized by red venous blood and the odor of bitter almonds

601. Exposure to this fungicide leads to increased hepatic weight

602. This agent acts by inhibiting acetylcholinesterase

603. This agent inhibits the inactivation of sodium channels

604. This agent causes convulsions by blocking the inhibitory neurotransmitter glycine

605. Poisoning with this agent is characterized initially by GI upset, but can lead to death by respiratory distress

DIRECTIONS (Questions 606–609): The group of questions below consists of four lettered headings followed by a list of numbered phrases or statements. For each numbered phrase or statement, select the **one** lettered heading that is most closely associated with it. Each heading may be used only once.

A. Aspirin
B. Tricyclic antidepressants
C. Acetaminophen
D. Benzodiazepines

606. Overdose results in hepatotoxicity because of the formation of a toxic metabolite

607. Overdose is characterized by antimuscarinic symptoms, such as tachycardia, dry mouth, and constipation

608. Overdose is the most common cause of reversible confusion in the elderly

609. Overdose is characterized by anion-gap metabolic acidosis

Toxicology

Answers and Discussion

582. B. Mercury exerts its toxic effects by binding to sulfhydryl groups and inhibiting cellular metabolism and function. (**Ref. 1,** p. 838; **Ref. 4,** p. 1599; **Ref. 12,** p. 896)

583. C. Exposure to arsenic can lead to peripheral neuropathy similar to that seen in Guillain-Barré syndrome, followed by increasing muscle weakness and eventual atrophy. (**Ref. 1,** p. 837; **Ref. 4,** p. 1603; **Ref. 12,** p. 895)

584. E. The distribution of lead in the body most closely resembles that of calcium. Its deposition in growing bones can be detected by x-ray studies and is used diagnostically in children. (**Ref. 1,** p. 834; **Ref. 4,** p. 1594; **Ref. 12,** pp. 892–893)

585. B. Lead has little effect on the pulmonary system. The primary effects of lead poisoning are seen in the GI, CNS, neuromuscular, renal, and hematological systems. (**Ref. 1,** p. 836; **Ref. 4,** pp. 1594–1595; **Ref. 12,** p. 894)

586. C. The earliest signs of iron poisoning are nausea, vomiting, and severe abdominal pain. These may be followed by cyanosis, drowsiness, and hyperventilation secondary to acidosis. (**Ref. 4,** p. 1291; **Ref. 12,** p. 496)

587. E. The administration of even therapeutic doses of opioids can cause constipation by decreasing peristaltic waves in the colon. To avoid this problem, laxatives or stool softeners are often given concurrently with opioids. (**Ref. 1**, p. 845; **Ref. 4**, p. 495; **Ref. 12**, p. 903)

588. D. Oral acetylcysteine acts to restore hepatic stores of glutathione depleted by acetaminophen. It is most effective when given within 10 hours of ingestion. (**Ref. 1**, p. 849; **Ref. 4**, p. 658; **Ref. 12**, p. 909)

589. E. Penicillamine forms complexes with lead that inhibit absorption and enhance excretion. (**Ref. 1**, p. 849; **Ref. 4**, p. 1610; **Ref. 12**, pp. 890–891)

590. B. Competitive inhibition of the metabolism of methanol to formaldehyde and formic acid is the basis for the administration of ethanol in methanol poisoning. Ethanol has a 100-fold greater affinity for the enzyme alcohol dehydrogenase than does methanol. (**Ref. 1**, p. 328; **Ref. 4**, p. 1624; **Ref. 12**, p. 358)

591. F. In iron poisoning, chelation therapy with IM or IV deferoxamine is the primary treatment aside from basic life-support measures. (**Ref. 1**, p. 834; **Ref. 4**, p. 1612; **Ref. 12**, p. 496)

592. C. Glucagon is used in the case of β-blocker toxicity because of its positive chronotropic and inotropic effects on the heart. (**Ref. 1**, p. 600; **Ref. 4**, p. 239; **Ref. 12**, p. 653)

593. A. Pralidoxime acts to reverse the effects of anticholinesterases by chemically reactivating the enzyme cholinesterase. (**Ref. 1**, p. 103; **Ref. 4**, p. 141; **Ref. 12**, p. 109)

594. D. The organs most affected by carbon monoxide poisoning are those most sensitive to oxygen deprivation, the brain and the heart. (**Ref. 1**, p. 824; **Ref. 4**, p. 1619; **Ref. 12**, pp. 881–882)

595. C. Initial exposure to carbon tetrachloride results in irritation to the eyes and other mucous membranes, dizziness, and nausea and vomiting. Continued exposure may result in coma, convulsions, and death. (**Ref. 1**, p. 825; **Ref. 4**, p. 1622; **Ref. 12**, p. 883)

596. B. Epidemiologic data support the connection between workers exposed to benzene and an increased incidence of leukemia. **(Ref. 1,** p. 826; **Ref. 4,** p. 1625; **Ref. 12,** pp. 883–884)

597. B. Methanol causes less inebriation than ethanol, and inebriation may not be an obvious sign of methanol poisoning unless very large quantities have been ingested. **(Ref. 1,** p. 328; **Ref. 4,** p. 1624; **Ref. 12,** p. 357)

598. E. Glycols have no effect on the hematopoietic system. Diagnosis is usually made by the presence of oxalate crystals in the urine and anion gap acidosis. **(Ref. 1,** p. 328; **Ref. 4,** p. 1625; **Ref. 12,** pp. 357–358)

599. A. Upon contact with mucous membranes, sulfur dioxide reacts to form sulfurous acid which is primarily responsible for the irritating effects this gas has on the respiratory tract. **(Ref. 1,** p. 824; **Ref. 4,** p. 1616; **Ref. 12,** p. 882)

600. B. Cyanide blocks the ability of the tissues to utilize oxygen carried in hemoglobin molecules. Thus, blood returning from the tissues is still rich in oxygen and retains its red color. **(Ref. 1,** p. 166; **Ref. 4,** p. 1630; **Ref. 12,** p. 176)

601. C. In addition to increasing hepatic weight, hexachlorobenzene increases the activity of the cytochrome P-450 system. **(Ref. 4,** p. 1635)

602. D. Organophosphates, such as malathion, inactivate acetylcholinesterase through a phosphorylation reaction. **(Ref. 1,** p. 827; **Ref. 4,** p. 140; **Ref. 12,** pp. 884–885)

603. F. The mechanism of action of DDT is not completely known, but it is believed to alter the transport of sodium and potassium across neuronal membranes, leading to repetitive or sustained muscle contractions. **(Ref. 1,** p. 826; **Ref. 4,** p. 1627; **Ref. 12,** p. 884)

604. E. Strychnine blocks the inhibitory effects of glycine in motor neurons, thus producing a characteristic seizure pattern in which antagonistic muscles simultaneously contract. **(Ref. 4,** p. 1632)

605. A. Initial symptoms of paraquat ingestion consist only of GI upset; however, the subsequent formation of free radicals and their effect on lung tissue leads to serious delayed pulmonary toxicity, which can be lethal. (**Ref. 1**, p. 829; **Ref. 4**, p. 1634; **Ref. 12**, p. 887)

606. C. Normally, acetaminophen is metabolized by glucuronidation and sulfation. When these pathways are saturated, the cytochrome P-450 system takes over and conjugates acetaminophen with hepatic stores of glutathione. Once these stores are depleted, accumulation of the toxic metabolite N-acetylbenzoiminoquinone leads to hepatic damage. (**Ref. 1**, p. 55; **Ref. 4**, p. 658; **Ref. 12**, pp. 54–55)

607. B. The anticholinergic effects associated with tricyclic antidepressant overdose include flushed dry skin, mydriasis, urinary retention, absent bowel sounds, dry mucosae, tachycardia, and arrhythmias. These symptoms may be life threatening, and the patient should be on cardiac and respiratory monitors. (**Ref. 1**, p. 845; **Ref. 4**, p. 413; **Ref. 12**, p. 903)

608. D. The high frequency with which benzodiazepines are prescribed for the elderly, along with decreased metabolic rate in this population, often results in acute toxic effects. The most common toxicities are confusion and drowsiness, which are often attributed to declining mental status rather than medications. (**Ref. 1**, p. 845; **Ref. 4**, p. 427; **Ref. 12**, pp. 337–338, 903)

609. A. Initial symptoms of aspirin overdose are tinnitus and GI upset. As the drug is further metabolized, more serious complications, such as acidosis and electrolyte imbalances, become increasingly life threatening. (**Ref. 1**, p. 845; **Ref. 4**, p. 651; **Ref. 12**, p. 903)

11

Drug Interactions

DIRECTIONS (Questions 610–630): Each of the questions or incomplete statements below is followed by five suggested answers or completions. Select the **one** that is best in each case.

---

610. Severe, prolonged alcohol abuse can lead to the abnormal metabolism of drugs because
   A. alcohol binds many compounds
   B. alcohol increases intestinal transit time
   C. prolonged use of alcohol damages the liver's ability to metabolize drugs
   D. alcohol desensitizes receptors to the effects of other medications
   E. the metabolism of such large quantities of alcohol uses up all available enzymes

611. Patients using theophylline should not smoke because
   A. smoking increases the metabolism of theophylline
   B. particles in cigarette and cigar smoke compete for binding sites in the lung with theophylline
   C. smoking irritates the lung and makes theophylline less effective
   D. theophylline enhances the effect of nicotine on the nervous system
   E. smoking inhibits metabolism of theophylline, thus increasing blood levels

612. β-Adrenergic blockers should be used with caution when given simultaneously with which of the following agents?
   A. Doxycycline
   B. Insulin
   C. Acetaminophen
   D. Fluoxetine
   E. Magnesium oxide

613. The mechanism of the interaction between antacids and ketoconazole is
   A. adsorption of ketoconazole to antacids
   B. increased metabolism of the antacid
   C. competition for binding sites
   D. increased GI pH inhibits absorption of ketoconazole
   E. increased emptying of gastric contents reduces activity of the antacid

614. Cimetidine decreases the metabolism of all of the following drugs EXCEPT
   A. lidocaine
   B. theophylline
   C. diazepam
   D. oral contraceptives
   E. ciprofloxacin

615. Patients taking monoamine oxidase inhibitors (MAOIs) should avoid cheese, red wines, and fermented meats because
   A. additive gastrointestinal irritation may occur
   B. these foods are high in tyramine
   C. these foods bind MAOIs in the GI tract
   D. MAOIs react with these foods to form toxic by-products
   E. MAOIs inhibit absorption of these foods

616. An increased incidence of cardiovascular incidents has been seen in patients who smoke and use
   A. oral contraceptives
   B. Potassium-sparing diuretics
   C. allopurinol
   D. class II antiarrhythmics
   E. albuterol

617. Phenylbutazone and tolbutamide should not be taken concurrently because
  A. the high sugar content of phenylbutazone requires higher doses of tolbutamide
  B. tolbutamide increases the metabolism of phenylbutazone
  C. phenylbutazone competes for binding sites with tolbutamide
  D. phenylbutazone inactivates proteins necessary for the absorption of tolbutamide
  E. tolbutamide binds phenylbutazone in the GI tract

618. Patients who consume alcohol while taking metronidazole can expect
  A. severe fatigue
  B. swelling of the extremities
  C. blurred vision
  D. severe nausea and vomiting
  E. diarrhea

619. Allopurinol should not be administered concurrently with mercaptopurine because
  A. additive mucositis occurs
  B. allopurinol inhibits the activity of mercaptopurine
  C. additive bone marrow toxicity develops
  D. mercaptopurine depletes uric acid
  E. allopurinol reacts with a metabolite of mercaptopurine

620. Patients taking warfarin should be advised to avoid green leafy vegetables because
  A. the green pigment interferes with warfarin metabolism
  B. they are rich in vitamin K
  C. they hinder dissolution of the warfarin tablet in the GI tract
  D. they contain proteins that compete with warfarin for binding sites
  E. the vegetables are undigestible when warfarin is present

621. Antacids have which of the following effects on antibiotics such as tetracycline?
  A. Increased metabolism
  B. Decreased absorption
  C. Decreased elimination
  D. Decreased metabolism
  E. Production of toxic by-products

622. Digitalis and diuretics should be carefully monitored when used concurrently because
   A. absorption of digitalis is decreased
   B. toxic metabolites accumulate
   C. dehydration is more likely
   D. potassium levels are decreased
   E. digitalis potentiates diuresis

623. Simultaneous use of lithium and diuretics is dangerous because of
   A. reduced clearance of lithium
   B. additive diuresis
   C. enhanced metabolism of lithium
   D. decreased clearance of diuretics
   E. accumulation of metabolites

624. The effect of simultaneous use of phenytoin and chloramphenicol is
   A. reduced antibacterial effect of chloramphenicol
   B. chelation of phenytoin
   C. decreased absorption of chloramphenicol
   D. development of a severe rash
   E. increased plasma concentration of phenytoin

625. Patients taking monoamine oxidase inhibitors should not take which of the following over-the-counter products without consulting their physician
   A. cold and allergy medications
   B. antidiarrheals
   C. aspirin-containing products
   D. topical antifungals
   E. creams containing hydrocortisone

626. Increased bleeding can occur when oral anticoagulants are given with
   A. barbiturates
   B. rifampin
   C. phenytoin
   D. furosemide
   E. aspirin

627. Amitriptyline should not be taken with which of the following drugs?
 A. Aspirin
 B. Chemotherapeutic agents
 C. Alcohol
 D. Cephalosporins
 E. Iron

628. Potentially toxic levels of this drug occur when given with erythromycin
 A. rifampin
 B. nystatin
 C. spironolactone
 D. acetaminophen
 E. theophylline

629. Beneficial drug interactions result from the concurrent use of local anesthetics with
 A. terfenadine
 B. phenytoin
 C. antidepressants
 D. epinephrine
 E. loperamide

630. β-Adrenergic blocking agents should not be used with
 A. verapamil
 B. acetaminophen
 C. bumetanide
 D. valproic acid
 E. diphenhydramine

Drug Interactions

Answers and Discussion

610. C. Prolonged use of alcohol damages the liver's ability to metabolize drugs. This can lead to increased blood levels of drugs or the accumulation of toxic metabolites. (**Ref. 1,** p. 932; **Ref. 4,** p. 373; **Ref. 12,** p. 988)

611. A. The increased metabolic rate associated with cigarette smoking is believed to be responsible for the increased clearance of theophylline in smokers. (**Ref. 1,** p. 942; **Ref. 4,** p. 627; **Ref. 10,** p. 2382; **Ref. 12,** p. 994)

612. B. β-Adrenergic blocking agents can block the symptoms of a hypoglycemic reaction to insulin, which can become life threatening if not treated. (**Ref. 1,** p. 935; **Ref. 4,** p. 239; **Ref. 12,** p. 990)

613. D. An acidic environment is required for the dissolution of ketoconazole; therefore, administration of antacids reduces dissolution, and subsequently absorption, of the drug. (**Ref. 1,** p. 933; **Ref. 4,** p. 1170; **Ref. 10,** p. 90; **Ref. 12,** p. 988)

614. E. Cimetidine has not been associated with any alteration in the activity of ciprofloxacin. (**Ref. 1,** p. 937; **Ref. 4,** p. 1059; **Ref. 10,** p. 1920; **Ref. 12,** p. 991)

615. B. Monoamine oxidase normally metabolizes tyramine. When this enzyme is inhibited, high levels of tyramine in the circulation can cause hypertension. (**Ref. 1**, p. 119; **Ref. 4**, p. 417; **Ref. 9**, p. 71; **Ref. 10**, p. 1379; **Ref. 12**, pp. 126–127)

616. A. There is a much higher risk of myocardial infarction in women taking oral contraceptives in general. This risk is further increased by smoking, age, and hypertension. (**Ref. 1**, pp. 573–574; **Ref. 4**, p. 1407; **Ref. 12**, pp. 622–623)

617. C. The effects of tolbutamide and other sulfonylureas are amplified during concurrent use of drugs such as phenylbutazone, dicumarol, and salicylates. (**Ref. 1**, p. 596; **Ref. 4**, p. 1486; **Ref. 10**, p. 1274; **Ref. 12**, p. 649)

618. D. Metronidazole inhibits alcohol dehydrogenase in a manner similar to that of disulfiram, causing severe nausea and vomiting, headache, and flushing when alcohol is consumed. (**Ref. 1**, p. 744; **Ref. 4**, p. 1004; **Ref. 10**, p. 543; **Ref. 12**, p. 800)

619. C. When allopurinol is given concurrently with mercaptopurine, the dose of mercaptopurine must be decreased by 25% in order to prevent toxicity. Allopurinol inhibits xanthine oxidase, the primary enzyme involved in the metabolism of mercaptopurine. (**Ref. 1**, p. 510; **Ref. 4**, p. 677; **Ref. 10**, p. 662; **Ref. 12**, p. 556)

620. B. Oral anticoagulants are antagonists of vitamin K, which is necessary in the activation of clotting factors II, VII, IX, X, and anticoagulant proteins C and S. Green leafy vegetables are high in vitamin K, and thus provide an alternative source for the activation of these factors and proteins. (**Ref. 1**, p. 468; **Ref 4**, pp. 1317–1320; **Ref. 12**, pp. 512–513)

621. B. Absorption of tetracyclines is impaired by concurrent ingestion of aluminum- and magnesium-containing antacids, dairy products, calcium, and bismuth subsalicylate. The mechanism of this interaction involves the chelation of the drug with divalent metal ions. (**Ref. 1**, p. 642; **Ref. 4**, p. 1119; **Ref. 10**, p. 332; **Ref. 12**, p. 696)

622. D. Concurrent use of digitalis and non–potassium-sparing diuretics must be carefully monitored. Hypokalemia secondary to diuretic use can lead to serious digitalis toxicity, manifested as cardiac arrhythmias. (**Ref. 1,** p. 183; **Ref. 4,** p. 834; **Ref. 10,** p. 953; **Ref. 12,** p. 991)

623. A. Clearance of lithium can be reduced as much as 25% when diuretics are being taken simultaneously. Dosage reductions are generally necessary in order to avoid lithium toxicity. (**Ref. 1,** p. 407; **Ref. 4,** p. 420; **Ref. 12,** p. 444)

624. E. Chloramphenicol, when administered with phenytoin, reduces the metabolism of phenytoin, leading to toxic side effects. (**Ref. 1,** p. 940; **Ref. 4,** p. 443; **Ref. 10,** p. 193; **Ref. 12,** p. 993)

625. A. Cough and cold preparations often contain drugs with sympathomimetic activity, such as pseudoephedrine, phenyl-propanolamine, and phenylephrine. Concurrent use of monoamine oxidase inhibitors with these agents can cause severe hypertension. (**Ref. 1,** p. 939; **Ref. 4,** p. 417; **Ref. 10,** p. 1380; **Ref. 12,** pp. 456–457)

626. E. Inhibition of platelet hemostasis associated with aspirin can lead to additive anticoagulant effects when taken with other oral anticoagulants. (**Ref. 1,** p. 470; **Ref. 4,** p. 647; **Ref. 12,** p. 514)

627. C. Sedative effects of all tricyclic antidepressants can be greatly potentiated by the concurrent use of alcohol. (**Ref. 1,** p. 417; **Ref. 4,** p. 413; **Ref. 10,** p. 1386; **Ref. 12,** p. 456)

628. E. Simultaneous administration of erythromycin and theophylline has resulted in several cases of severe theophylline toxicity. (**Ref. 1,** p. 942; **Ref. 4,** p. 1133; **Ref. 10,** pp. 198–199; **Ref. 12,** p. 994)

629. D. Local anesthetics are commonly combined with epinephrine because the vasoconstrictive effect of the epinephrine slows anesthetic absorption. (**Ref. 1,** p. 364; **Ref. 4,** pp. 316–317; **Ref. 10,** pp. 772–773; **Ref. 12,** p. 397)

630. A. Concurrent use of verapamil and β-adrenergic blockers has been associated with significant bradycardia or AV block. (**Ref. 4,** p. 870; **Ref. 10,** p. 1077)

12

Problem-Related Questions

DIRECTIONS (Questions 631–700): Each section below consists of a problem followed by a series of questions. Each of the questions or incomplete statements is followed by five suggested answers or completions. Select the **one** that is best in each case.

Questions 631–634: Select the single best answer from the choices provided.

Mrs Broncho suffered from a severe allergy to peanuts and carried an auto-injector of epinephrine for emergencies. After ingesting some peanuts in a cookie, she felt her chest tightening and reached into her purse for her medication only to find that the needle injected a dose into her thumb. Her thumb became numb and blanched. She thought this was a response to histamine as a consequence of the needle stick and decided to take an antihistamine. When her condition did not improve she came to the emergency room at a local hospital.

631. The reaction Mrs Broncho experienced was due to
   A. intense vasodilation draining the thumb
   B. β_2-adrenergic receptor activation
   C. histamine release
   D. an axon reflex
   E. α_1-adrenergic receptor-induced vasoconstriction

632. Pharmacologic management of this condition would be
   A. administration of glucocorticoids orally
   B. administration of glucocorticoids parenterally
   C. infiltration of phentolamine into the thumb
   D. topical use of a local anesthetic
   E. injection of nitroprusside

633. The effects of histamine on blood vessels would be
   A. vasoconstriction through α-receptors
   B. vasoconstriction through H_2-receptors
   C. vasoconstriction through D_1-receptors
   D. vasodilation through β_2-receptors
   E. vasodilation through H_1-receptors

634. Glucocorticoids
   A. cause vasodilation
   B. antagonize adrenergic vasoconstriction
   C. cause up-regulation of β-adrenergic receptors
   D. would constrict blood vessels if administered systemically
   E. augment the action of histamine

Questions 635–636: Jim had just turned 12. He has a five-year history of epilepsy, which was well controlled with phenytoin. Within the last year, Jim has had an increase in seizure activity and his parents have decided to have his condition evaluated.

635. Increased seizure activity is most likely the result of which of the following?
   A. Decreased compliance
   B. Loss of effectiveness of phenytoin
   C. The need to add a second agent
   D. Fetal hydantoin syndrome
   E. The development of toxicity associated with puberty

636. Assuming that the levels of phenytoin were in the therapeutic range, what might explain the lack of effectiveness?
   A. The development of a second seizure type
   B. A decreased activity of P-450
   C. Decreased binding to plasma proteins
   D. Autostimulation of its own metabolism
   E. An increase in the half-life of phenytoin

Questions 637–638: A college student participating in a football rally decides to ignite the bonfire by throwing gasoline on the haystack, which is smoldering. It is moist from a recent rain. He trips and spills the gasoline, which explosively ignites, trapping him in the flames. He is brought to the emergency room and a neuromuscular blocker is to be administered.

637. Which of the following considerations is correct?
   A. A centrally-acting agent should be selected
   B. A college age student would be expected to have a decreased renal clearance of neuromuscular blockers
   C. Burned patients are resistant to nondepolarizing agents
   D. Increased levels of neuromuscular blockers will be needed due to their antagonism of general anesthetic agents
   E. Succinylcholine may cause hypokalemia in this patient

638. In a burned patient
   A. increased acetylcholine release would be expected
   B. aminoglycosides would potentiate neuromuscular blockade
   C. depolarizing blocking agents would augment nondepolarizing blockers
   D. acetylcholinesterase inhibitors would potentiate nondepolarizing blockers
   E. calcium channel blockers would inhibit neuromuscular blockade

Questions 639–641: A neighbor of yours has knocked on the door because he was out walking and began to experience angina pectoris. He said he takes a long-acting nitrate ester, but it seems to be ineffective.

639. All of the following statements are true EXCEPT
   A. nitroglycerin is usually administered sublingually
   B. transdermal nitroglycerin provides prophylactic therapy for angina pectoris
   C. sublingual nitroglycerin is usually effective within 2 to 5 minutes
   D. long-acting nitrates apparently saturate hepatic nitrate reductase
   E. nitroglycerin ointment can be used to reduce the development of tolerance

238 / 12: Problem-Related Questions

640. Nitroglycerin
   A. may cause rebound hypertension if use is discontinued
   B. causes relaxation of vascular smooth muscle by reducing cytosolic free Ca^{++}
   C. is not effective if taken shortly before exercise
   D. reduces the production of NO
   E. exerts its main action on resistance vessels

641. Other pharmacologic approaches to the treatment of angina pectoris include
   A. β-Adrenergic blocking agents
   B. serotonin
   C. thromboxane
   D. norepinephrine
   E. ergot alkaloids

Questions 642–644: Mr Mood Disorder has been taking a tricyclic antidepressant; however, he is experiencing a considerable number of side effects. He wishes to make a change and has come seeking information on other agents.

642. The common side effects of tricyclic antidepressants include
   A. weight loss
   B. bradycardia
   C. increased salivation
   D. urinary retention
   E. diarrhea

643. He has heard of a new compound called fluoxetine, which he refers to as Prozac, and is interested in its side effects. You inform him that it causes all of the following EXCEPT
   A. anxiety
   B. ejaculatory delay
   C. diarrhea
   D. anticholinergic effects
   E. some minor weight loss

644. Mr Disorder is curious about how these compounds act and wants to know about the mechanism of action. He is informed that fluoxetine
   A. acts by inhibiting catecholamine and serotonin uptake.
   B. is a selective serotonin reuptake inhibitor

C. inhibits MAO
D. blocks postsynaptic serotonin receptors
E. inhibits dopamine uptake

Questions 645–646: Edward, a 51-year-old man weighing approximately 65 kg, after consuming several bottles of beer during the course of an evening, drank the entire contents of two 8-ounce bottles of an adult liquid pain reliever, called drug A, at about 10 PM. At breakfast time, around 8 AM the following day, he experienced anorexia, nausea, vomiting, and abdominal pain. At the insistence of his wife, he agreed to see a physician. A serum assay revealed a plasma concentration of drug A greater than 70 µg/mL. A 5% solution of drug B was given as a loading dose of 180 mL (140 mg/kg). The patient was then admitted to the hospital, where administration of drug B was continued in doses of 90 mL of the 5% solution at 4-hour intervals until assays indicated that drug A concentration in plasma was below hepatotoxic levels.

645. Drug A, the agent producing the toxic effects, was
A. sodium salicylate
B. acetylcysteine
C. colchicine
D. acetaminophen
E. sulfinpyrazone

646. Drug B, the agent used to antagonize the toxic effects of drug A, was
A. sodium salicylate
B. acetylcysteine
C. colchicine
D. acetaminophen
E. sulfinpyrazone

Questions 647–648: Mrs Nextdoor rings your doorbell and asks you to drive to the local pharmacy to pick up medications the pediatrician has called in for her son, who has asthma. She tells you he has had a cold the last few days and has started to wheeze. She reminds you that he is allergic to penicillin. As you start to back out of the driveway, she hands you his cromolyn metered-dose inhaler and asks that you refill this as well, since he really needs his inhaler. You are a considerate neighbor and do as she asks and return with sustained-action theophylline capsules, erythromycin, and a cromolyn metered-dose inhaler.

647. The pediatrician has probably ordered erythromycin because
  A. it's one of the best tolerated antibiotics and will cause little GI upset
  B. patients with penicillin allergy are less likely to exhibit cross-sensitivity to erythromycin than to synthetic penicillins or cephalosporin
  C. erythromycin will not interact with the child's maintenance medications, theophylline and cromolyn
  D. the cold is probably viral
  E. erythromycin has a narrow spectrum of activity

648. The pharmacist asked you to tell Mrs Nextdoor that cromolyn is ineffective in treating acute episodes of asthma. A better choice would have been
  A. short-duration inhaled β-agonist bronchodilator for wheezing
  B. an inhaled corticosteroid for inflammation
  C. a short-term oral steroid "burst"
  D. a long-duration inhaled β-agonist for nighttime use
  E. all of the above

Questions 649–650: While at home for the holidays, you hear your aunt tell your mother that she thinks she has a urinary tract infection because she finds she is urinating with greater and greater frequency. You remember that she is a non–insulin-dependent diabetic who also has hypertension, and you notice that she has gained a considerable amount of weight since you last saw her. Since she knows you have just completed your pharmacology course, she tells you that her current medications are glyburide for her diabetes and propranolol and hydrochlorothiazide for her hypertension. She is proud of her new glucometer, and takes her morning readings. They have been in the 250 to 300 range all of this week.

649. A possible cause for her increased urinary frequency is
  A. a urinary tract infection
  B. it may be a symptom of uncontrolled hyperglycemia
  C. the thiazide diuretic that she takes for hypertension
  D. increased fluid intake
  E. all of the above

650. A possible cause for the elevated blood glucose levels she finds is
  A. her recent weight gain
  B. the β-blocker that her doctor has prescribed

C. the hydrochlorothiazide she takes daily
D. a urinary tract infection
E. all of the above

Questions 651–653: Approximately two years ago, Mrs Sweetblood was diagnosed with non–insulin-dependent diabetes. For the past year, she has had difficulty sleeping and decreased libido. She was started on amitriptyline six months ago and is sleeping better, but has noticed an increase in appetite and has gained approximately 20 pounds. She feels too tired to go to the mall to walk every morning, a practice she had followed regularly. Her blood glucose levels, which had been reasonably well controlled, are increasing gradually. On her last visit, her doctor discontinued her amitriptyline and started her on fluoxetine.

651. Her gradual increase in blood glucose levels is probably due to
  A. weight gain and decreased exercise level caused by amitriptyline
  B. amitriptyline-induced decrease in oral hypoglycemic absorption
  C. decreased glucose metabolism due to tricyclic antidepressants
  D. tricyclic antidepressant-induced craving for sweets
  E. all of the above

652. Other side effects of tricyclic antidepressants include
  A. blurred vision
  B. orthostatic hypotension
  C. constipation
  D. palpitations
  E. all of the above

653. Fluoxetine may be a better antidepressant choice for this patient because
  A. it is more sedating than amitriptyline and less likely to cause agitation
  B. it does not cause weight gain and may cause slight weight loss in some patients
  C. it is less expensive than amitriptyline
  D. it is less likely to cause disturbances in sexual function
  E. all of the above

Questions 654–658: Mr Weekend Athlete has injured a leg in a "pick-up" football game. He is in severe and constant pain, which was not relieved by medications he purchased at the drug store. Examination reveals that no bones are broken. Something is needed for pain relief.

654. Mr Athlete asks you for hydromorphone because it is a potent agent. He is informed that
  A. hydromorphone is a better agent since it is more potent than morphine
  B. equianalgesic doses are equieffective
  C. hydromorphone is more apt to cause respiratory depression
  D. aspirin would be more effective for this type of pain
  E. take all of this prescription for 100 hydromorphone tablets

655. Mr Athlete tells you that he feels strange when taking this drug (hydromorphone). He knows it is for pain but he does not understand what is happening to him. You explain that
  A. he need not be concerned, because the opioid he is taking does not cause dependence
  B. opioids block receptors in the brain to cause pain relief
  C. he needs to switch to a different opioid
  D. opioid analgesics should not be used for chronic pain
  E. the opioid blocks the emotional response to pain but he may still identify the pain stimulus

656. On day two, you learn that Mr Athlete called the office and asked the nurse if it was all right for his mother to use this prescription for a cough. After telling him that it is illegal to transfer this medication to another person, you inform him that
  A. meperidine is a better agent for cough, since it is less potent
  B. it would be a good agent to relieve the cough
  C. she should take dextromethorphan
  D. propoxyphene is preferred for cough
  E. naloxone should be used

657. Four days later, Mr Athlete telephones your office to inform you that his prescription has been used and that his pain is much better. His leg is swollen and sensitive to touch. He is advised
  A. to take an NSAID such as aspirin or ibuprofen
  B. to use acetaminophen, since it will cause less gastric irritation

C. that he should get another prescription for the opioid
D. that the chronic pain needs a different type of therapy
E. that a drug that activates mu receptors should be tried

658. Mr Athlete also heard that these opioid agents are good for diarrhea, and asks about this use. He is informed that
A. this is correct and it is an appropriate use of opioids if needed
B. he should not use opioids, but should take diphenoxylate instead
C. NSAIDs would be more effective
D. an antagonist of mu receptors would still be effective on smooth muscle
E. acetaminophen should be used

Questions 659–663: Mrs A has recently been diagnosed with breast cancer. In discussing her treatment options with her, her physician tells her there are several drugs used in the treatment of breast cancer.

659. All of the following are potential treatments EXCEPT
A. CMF (cyclophosphamide, methotrexate, and 5-fluorouracil)
B. lomustine
C. paclitaxel
D. megestrol acetate
E. CAF (cyclophosphamide, doxorubicin, and 5-fluorouracil)

660. Mrs A says that she has heard of the drug paclitaxel but has also heard that there are some severe side-effects associated with its use. Dr Chemo informs her that one of the most serious side effects associated with the administration of paclitaxel is
A. nausea and vomiting
B. hypertension
C. hematuria
D. hypersensitivity reaction
E. phlebitis and irritation at the injection site

661. Since she is afraid of needles, Mrs A wants to know if there are any oral medications available. Dr Chemo tells her that antiestrogens have been used in the treatment of breast cancer. Which of the following drugs might be used for this purpose?
   A. Medroxyprogesterone
   B. Cyclophosphamide
   C. Methotrexate
   D. Leucovorin
   E. Tamoxifen

662. Mrs A is concerned about the nausea and vomiting often associated with chemotherapy. She wants to know what agents are available for the treatment of this condition. Dr Chemo tells her that all of the following are used in the treatment of chemotherapy-induced nausea and vomiting EXCEPT
   A. prochlorperazine
   B. dimenhydrinate
   C. ondansetron
   D. lorazepam
   E. dexamethasone

663. Prior to receiving chemotherapy, Mrs A begins to exhibit signs of hypercalcemia. Dr Chemo assures her that this is common in breast cancer patients and is treated with all of the following EXCEPT
   A. calcitonin
   B. vitamin D
   C. hydration
   D. furosemide
   E. bisphosphonates

Questions 664–667: Mrs Pregnant is in the latter part of the second trimester. She comes in for an evaluation and is found to have dangerously high blood pressure. She needs some control, but is complaining about edema. Can something be done to relieve the pressure? She has many questions about taking drugs and what effect they will have on the baby. In response to her questions you provide answers to assist her in understanding how drugs work.

664. The edema in the above case should be
   A. aggressively managed
   B. treated with loop diuretics

C. treated with thiazides
D. observed and treated only if problems develop
E. reduced with a benign agent like mannitol

665. When is it most dangerous to take drugs during pregnancy?
A. At term
B. During the second trimester
C. During the first trimester
D. While trying to get pregnant
E. Drugs and pregnancy pose no concerns

666. The FDA provides classification of drug safety during pregnancy. An example of one of these categories is
A. Class A—well-controlled studies fail to indicate a risk
B. Class B—animal studies have not been done
C. Class C—well-controlled human studies demonstrate a risk
D. Class D—studies have not been done
E. Class X—exempt from classification

667. Near the end of her pregnancy she develops premature contractions. All of the following might be trial medications EXCEPT
A. magnesium salts intravenously
B. terbutaline
C. ritodrine
D. ethanol
E. oxytocin

Questions 668–670: After watching your friend Tubby consume 50 chicken wings and two baskets of fries, you suggest that he might want to get his cholesterol levels tested. Heeding your expert medical advice, he does so and finds the following results: increased triglycerides and increased LDL.

668. You suggest the following initial therapy
A. angioplasty
B. nicotinic acid
C. a bile acid sequestrant
D. a change in diet and exercise
E. a fibric acid derivative

669. After months of attempting to diet, Tubby just can't stay away from those Big Macs, and his triglyceride and LDL levels have not changed. You suggest initiation of drug therapy with niacin, which works by
A. increasing the activity of lipoprotein lipase
B. inhibiting the resorption of cholesterol
C. inhibition of VLDL secretion, in turn decreasing production of LDL
D. inhibition of HMG-CoA reductase
E. binding intestinal bile acids

670. After several weeks on niacin therapy, Tubby complains that he is experiencing flushing after each dose. You suggest that this can be reduced by
A. taking aspirin one-half hour prior to the niacin
B. taking the niacin with food
C. taking the niacin all in one dose at bedtime
D. decreasing the interval between doses
E. decreasing the dose

Questions 671–674: Mr Runnynose, a patient you saw yesterday for treatment of an upper respiratory infection, calls to ask your recommendation of an antihistamine.

671. You ask him what symptoms he is attempting to treat, because antihistamines are used in all of the following conditions EXCEPT
A. sinus congestion
B. allergic rhinitis
C. motion sickness
D. Parkinson's disease
E. insomnia

672. Mr Runnynose explains that he has had a runny nose and watery eyes and would like you to recommend a product that produces minimal sedation. You recommend
A. dimenhydrinate
B. clemastine
C. diphenhydramine
D. phenylpropanolamine
E. doxylamine

673. Mr Runnynose says that he has heard of a prescription antihistamine called Seldane that causes no sedation. You explain to him that this would not be a good choice for him because of a potential interaction with which of the following drugs?
  A. Astemizole
  B. Propranolol
  C. Cimetidine
  D. Erythromycin
  E. Cephalexin

674. While you are explaining how antihistamines work by blocking histamine receptors, Mr Runnynose asks if there are any drugs available that block the release of histamine. You answer that there is one such drug
  A. loratadine
  B. meclizine
  C. cromolyn
  D. famotidine
  E. diphenhydramine

Questions 675–678: Mr Hyper Tension, a 40-year-old white male, has been experiencing headaches, pounding in his chest, and excessive sweating when he runs early in the morning. He claims that this has been getting progressively worse over the last year. On examination you find he has a blood pressure of 140/100, which is confirmed on repeated testing.

675. In considering essential hypertension
  A. it is due to altered autonomic nervous system function
  B. increased cardiac output is usually observed
  C. the renin-angiotensin-aldosterone system is the cause
  D. there is no specific cause
  E. a brain tumor is most often the predisposing factor

676. Antihypertensive agents act through all of the following anatomic control sites EXCEPT
  A. kidneys
  B. intestine
  C. heart
  D. brain
  E. blood vessels

677. Drug therapy usually includes an agent or agents from any of the following drug classes EXCEPT
   A. cardiac glycosides
   B. diuretics
   C. direct vasodilators
   D. angiotensin-converting-enzyme inhibitors
   E. sympathetic-nervous-system–blocking agents

678. Mr Tension knows of friends who take propranolol and wants to know how it acts. You tell him that propranolol
   A. stimulates the heart to move blood through constricted vessels
   B. is a vasodilator
   C. causes CNS stimulation, which lowers blood pressure
   D. removes excess fluid from the body
   E. inhibits renin release

Questions 679–683: Ms Intoxicated is a sophomore college student who is pledging a sorority. She was at a local bar and was challenged by her boyfriend to see who could drink the most. Egged on by a group of students, she drank 15 one-ounce shots before she collapsed on the floor. She was taken to the emergency room where she was diagnosed with acute alcohol intoxication.

679. Which of the following facts about ethanol is true?
   A. It is primarily metabolized by the P-450 system
   B. Gastric alcohol dehydrogenase is lower in women than men
   C. Acetaldehyde has accumulated in this patient
   D. Alcohol is slowly absorbed from the GI tract
   E. Ingested alcohol is mainly excreted unchanged

680. Ms Intoxicated is an Oriental; thus she
   A. metabolizes ethanol more rapidly
   B. has a greater level of microsomal oxidase activity
   C. has less acetaldehyde dehydrogenase activity
   D. has the same metabolism of ethanol as anyone else
   E. metabolized ethanol to methanol

681. The laboratory report shows that the blood alcohol is 250 mg/dL. The therapy for acute ethanol intoxication is
   A. pump the stomach
   B. maintain respiratory and cardiovascular function

C. administer disulfiram
D. administer fructose
E. give an analeptic

682. The boyfriend informs you that Ms Intoxicated has been treated at the student health service and you are concerned because of a drug interaction. All of the following are of concern EXCEPT
A. cephalosporins
B. acetaminophen
C. metronidazole
D. propoxyphene
E. hydrochlorothiazide

Questions 683–685: Carrie Coed started to take her roommate's thyroid medication to combat the "freshman 15" (weight gain often seen the first year in college). She feels nervous and jittery and goes to the student health center.

683. Adverse effects of unneeded thyroid hormone (T_4) are similar to the symptoms of thyroid hyperactivity and include all but
A. tremor
B. nervousness and anxiety
C. dry skin
D. muscle weakness
E. eyelid lag and retraction

684. The preparation of choice in the treatment of hypothyroidism is
A. levothyroxine
B. liothyronine
C. desiccated thyroid
D. methimazole
E. propylthiouracil

685. The symptoms for which her roommate's doctor prescribed thyroid hormone include
A. lethargy
B. decreased basal metabolic rate
C. stiffness, muscle fatigue
D. decreased urination
E. all of the above

Questions 686–690: Mrs Hefty told the ladies in her creative cooking class that her husband was less and less willing to eat the new foods she was cooking. He said they aggravated his ulcers and kept him from sleeping at night because he had such terrible heartburn. She bought him a large bottle of antacid tablets because he was using up all her baking soda trying to relieve his indigestion.

686. The following is (are) true concerning the use of sodium bicarbonate for indigestion
  A. large amounts of CO_2 are produced, causing flatulence and belching
  B. $NaHCO_3$ is almost completely absorbed from the tract and large doses cause transient metabolic alkalosis
  C. antacids should be administered 1/2 to 1 hour after meals
  D. large doses of $NaHCO_3$ can actually increase the amount of acid Mr Hefty's stomach secretes after a meal
  E. all of the above

687. The actions of metoclopramide include all of the following EXCEPT
  A. accelerated gastric emptying
  B. reduced reflux from duodenum and stomach into esophagus
  C. increased jejunal peristalsis
  D. decreased gastric secretion
  E. overcoming of gastric stasis of diabetic neuropathy

688. Which of the following statement(s) is (are) true concerning antacids?
  A. Magnesium (Mg^{2+})-containing products cause constipation
  B. Calcium carbonate products are similar in effect to sodium bicarbonate
  C. Aluminum (Al^{3+}) products cause diarrhea
  D. Al^{3+} products are indicated as a major method of decreasing intestinal absorption of phosphate in uremic patients
  E. Thiazide diuretics can be used to increase Ca^{2+} elimination when necessary

689. Mr Hefty asked his doctor to give him something to help eliminate his heartburn and was told
  A. to sleep without a pillow to alleviate his distress
  B. to take a large dose of $NaHCO_3$ at bedtime
  C. to ask his wife to quit her cooking class

D. to take metoclopramide before meals and at bedtime
E. to take his antacid tablets or sodium bicarbonate with milk or cream

690. An alternative treatment the doctor suggested was ranitidine twice daily. All of the following are side-effects of ranitidine EXCEPT
A. headaches
B. dizziness and nausea
C. myalgia
D. bezoar formation
E. tinnitus

Questions 691–696: Mr Abnormal Rhythm is a third-year medical student who is putting in long hours on his clerkship. He drinks coffee on a continuous basis. He has been experiencing episodes of rapid heart rate, and he notices extrasystoles occurring periodically. Being a newly proclaimed expert in cardiology, he begins to analyze his problem. He is deciding what to do to eliminate the abnormal rhythm. He is an older student at age 35 and has had some problems with his prostate.

691. Mr Rhythm first reviews mechanisms of arrhythmia production and realizes arrhythmias can be suppressed by agents that
A. increase dV/dt in phase 4
B. decrease the refractory period in ventricular muscle
C. decrease resting membrane potential
D. increase AV conduction
E. increase vagal tone

692. The best advice his classmates give Mr Rhythm is that he
A. should decrease coffee drinking
B. should get some rest and not be concerned
C. has paroxysmal atrial tachycardia
D. should suppress the extrasystoles
E. has a reversible arrhythmia that needs drug treatment

693. If drug therapy was instituted, which of the following agents would be contraindicated for Mr Rhythm?
A. Verapamil
B. Disopyramide
C. Propranolol
D. Digitalis
E. Nadolol

694. Classification of antiarrhythmic agents includes all of the following EXCEPT
   A. calcium channel blockers
   B. sodium channel blockers
   C. agents that prolong the action-potential duration
   D. agents that decrease vagal tone
   E. β-adrenergic blocking agents

695. Mr Rhythm is correctly informed by his friends that
   A. arrhythmias are dangerous and should be treated
   B. modern drug therapy is relatively safe
   C. most antiarrhythmic agents are not toxic
   D. antiarrhythmic agents cause arrhythmias
   E. the Cardiac Arrhythmia Supression Test (CAST) demonstrated that the newer lidocaine-like agents decrease cardiovascular mortality

696. Assuming that Mr Rhythm has a supraventricular tachycardia needing treatment, the most appropriate agent would most likely be
   A. quinidine
   B. verapamil
   C. bretylium
   D. flecainide
   E. procainamide

Questions 697–700: At your high school reunion, you spend some time talking to Ms Spacey, your sophomore English teacher. You remember that she has always been frail and recall that she suffered a mild stroke last year. She now has an upper-respiratory infection, and seems congested. You offer to get her some punch, and she declines, saying that her stomach hurts, and she has coughed up some blood. Knowing you are in medical school, she shows you her medications: sodium warfarin, which she has taken daily since her stroke, and trimethoprim-sulfamethoxazole, which she has taken for the past week to treat her cold.

697. Trimethoprim-sulfamethoxazole may be a problem, because
   A. it causes photosensitivity, and Ms Spacey will be unable to attend the outdoor picnic tomorrow
   B. it causes GI upset
   C. it prohibits metabolism of her anticoagulant to increase prothrombin time

D. sulfonamides can precipitate in urine, causing crystalluria if Ms Spacey does not increase her fluid intake during treatment

E. all of the above

698. Other medications Ms Spacey should avoid include
A. antidiabetic agents
B. aspirin
C. third-generation cephalosporins
D. barbiturates
E. all of the above

699. Ms Spacey will see her doctor for treatment of her GI bleeding. The doctor should not prescribe
A. aluminum hydroxide/magnesium hydroxide
B. sucralfate
C. cimetidine
D. calcium carbonate
E. any of the above

700. Anticoagulant therapy is indicated for all but
A. preventions of thromboembolism
B. transient ischemic attacks
C. prophylaxis of myocardial reinfarction
D. prophylaxis and treatment of deep vein thrombosis
E. duodenal ulcers

Problem-Related Questions

Answers and Discussion

631. E. The injection of epinephrine into a digit, where the main effect would be activation of α_1-adrenergic receptor activation, may result in intense vasoconstriction. If blood flow were obstructed by initial vasoconstriction at the base of the digit, the effect would be long lasting. There is a potential to completely inhibit perfusion of the tissue. (**Ref. 1,** p. 114; **Ref. 4,** pp. 198–199; **Ref. 12,** p. 121)

632. C. The only specific antagonist of the α-adrenergic effects of epinephrine is phentolamine. It is indicated for infiltration into the digit, thus relieving the vasoconstriction. It may be used to antagonize the effect of adrenergic vasoconstriction when extravasation occurs. (**Ref. 1,** p. 125; **Ref. 4,** p. 225; **Ref. 12,** p. 134)

633. E. Histamine causes vasodilation through both H_1- and H_2-receptors since the use of classical H_1 antihistamines with H_2-receptor blockers more effectively inhibits vasodilation. (**Ref. 1,** p. 231; **Ref. 4,** p. 580; **Ref. 12,** p. 253)

634. C. Glucocorticoids are often employed for their anti-inflammatory effect and they do have direct effects on blood vessels. The most correct answer, however, is that glucocorticoids will cause up-regulation of adrenergic receptors. (**Ref. 1,** pp. 545–546; **Ref. 4,** p. 634; **Ref. 12,** p. 594)

254

635. A. When children approach the teenage years, compliance is often decreased, since the taking of this medication still has a stigma associated with it. Plasma levels should be monitored. (**Ref. 1,** p. 346; **Ref. 4,** p. 457; **Ref. 12,** pp. 439, 457)

636. A. An attempt to identify or reclassify the correct seizure pattern is the most likely of the choices presented. Autostimulation of its own metabolism is unlikely for phenytoin. Decreased P-450 activity, decreased binding to plasma proteins, and an increase in half-life would all lead to increased levels of phenytoin. (**Ref. 1,** pp. 334–335, 345; **Ref. 4,** pp. 440, 456; **Ref. 12,** pp. 364–365)

637. C. The resistance of burned patients to neuromuscular blocking agents is thought to be due to a proliferation of extrajunctional receptors. Increased toxicity of or sensitivity to neuromuscular blocking agents is usually associated with decreased renal clearance in the elderly. Centrally-acting agents are inappropriate. Burned patients have hyperkalemia. General anesthetics usually potentiate neuromuscular blockade. (**Ref. 1,** pp. 378–379; **Ref. 2,** pp. 175–176, 290; **Ref. 12,** p. 414)

638. B. Aminoglycoside antibiotics potentiate the effect of neuromuscular blocking agents. Neostigmine would inhibit nondepolarizing blockers. Calcium channel blockers potentiate both depolarizing and nondepolarizing neuromuscular blockers. (**Ref. 1,** p. 378; **Ref. 4,** p. 175; **Ref. 12,** p. 414)

639. E. Chronic or repeated use of organic nitrates results in tolerance. Intermittent use is an important factor in maintaining effectiveness of nitroglycerin. (**Ref. 1,** pp. 166–167; **Ref. 2,** pp. 268–269; **Ref. 4,** pp. 769–770; **Ref. 12,** pp. 176–177)

640. B. Nitroglycerin acts to release nitric oxide, leading to increased cGMP levels and decreased cytosolic calcium ion. Its primary effect in low doses is to relieve preload by relaxing capacitance vessels. It can be taken prophylactically to prevent exercise-induced angina. (**Ref. 1,** pp. 164, 167; **Ref. 2,** pp. 267–268; **Ref. 4,** pp. 766, 768; **Ref. 12,** pp. 174, 176)

641. A. All of the agents listed except β-blockers have the potential to induce coronary artery vasospasm and this causes angina pectoris.

The β-adrenergic blocking agents decrease cardiac inotropic and chronotropic activity due to sympathetic nervous system activation. (**Ref. 2**, pp. 267, 271–272; **Ref. 12**, p. 182)

642. **D.** Side effects of TCA drugs are typically the opposite of those listed. Weight gain, cardiac arrhythmias (tachycardia), dry mouth, and constipation occur. (**Ref. 1**, p. 417; **Ref. 2**, p. 401; **Ref. 4**, p. 411; **Ref. 12**, p. 457)

643. **D.** Fluoxetine does not cause the anticholinergic and cardiovascular side effects observed with tricyclic antidepressants. (**Ref. 1**, p. 413; **Ref. 2**, p. 405; **Ref. 4**, p. 406; **Ref. 12**, p. 453)

644. **B.** Fluoxetine is an SSRI. The other mechanisms listed are proposed for iproniazid (MAOI) imipramine (inhibits catecholamine and serotonin reuptake), trazodone (blocks postsynaptic serotonin receptors and bupropion (inhibits dopamine uptake). (**Ref. 1**, p. 413; **Ref. 2**, p. 403; **Ref. 4**, pp. 406, 408, 411, 415; **Ref. 12**, p. 453)

645. **D.** Hepatotoxicity may follow ingestion of a single dose of 10 to 15 g of acetaminophen. This toxic effect has been attributed to a metabolite that binds to cellular constituents, particularly glutathione. When production of the toxic metabolite exceeds the quantity of glutathione available for its inactivation, hepatotoxicity occurs. (**Ref. 1**, p. 506; **Ref. 2**, pp. 436–437; **Ref. 4**, p. 658; **Ref. 12**, p. 552)

646. **B.** Acetylcysteine is a sulfhydryl compound that probably acts, in part, by replenishing hepatic stores of glutathione. It has been shown to be effective if given less than 24 hours after acetaminophen overdose. (**Ref. 1**, p. 499; **Ref. 2**, pp. 436–437; **Ref. 4**, p. 658; **Ref. 12**, p. 552)

647. **B.** Erythromycin is a broad spectrum antibiotic frequently used for patients intolerant of penicillin. Anorexia, nausea, vomiting, abdominal cramping, and diarrhea sometimes result from oral administration. Erythromycin reduces the clearance of theophylline and concomitant use can result in theophylline toxicity. (**Ref. 1**, pp. 684, 685; **Ref. 4**, p. 627; **Ref. 12**, pp. 740–741).

648. E. Cromolyn, as well as nedocromil, is indicated for prophylaxis of asthma and not for exacerbations. Inhaled corticosteroid or oral steroid bursts with inhaled bronchodilator as needed for wheezing are the current National Asthma Education Program recommendations. (**Ref. 2**, pp. 510–511; **Ref. 4**, pp. 632–635; **Ref. 12**, pp. 317–318).

649. E. Thiazides, which are used to treat edema as well as hypertension, act at the distal convoluted tubule to produce diuresis. Each of the other choices can also be true. (**Ref. 1**, pp 219–221; **Ref. 4**, p. 786; **Ref. 12**, p. 239)

650. E. Obesity is a common risk factor for diabetes mellitus. Infections can bring about elevated blood glucose levels. Thiazide diuretics and β-blockers both impair carbohydrate tolerance. (**Ref. 1**, pp. 221, 586–587, 594; **Ref. 4**, pp. 233, 787; **Ref. 12**, pp. 120, 240, 637)

651 A. A common undesired effect of tricyclic antidepressants is weight gain due to increased appetite and sedation, which decreases physical activity. Increased body weight decreases carbohydrate tolerance. (**Ref. 1**, p. 417; **Ref. 4**, p. 787; **Ref. 12**, p. 457)

652. E. Tricyclic antidepressants cause many anticholinergic and cardiovascular side effects, such as blurred vision, constipation, urinary retention, palpitation, and orthostatic hypotension. (**Ref. 1**, pp. 401, 405, 417; **Ref. 2**, p. 401; **Ref. 12**, p. 457)

653. B. Fluoxetine, a selective serotonin reuptake inhibitor, does not cause weight increase. A modest weight reduction may be seen in some patients early in therapy, but weight loss does not continue with chronic use. It is not indicated for weight loss in obesity. (**Ref. 6**, pp. 401, 405; **Ref. 12**, p. 457)

654. B. In equieffective doses (in this case, equianalgesic doses), the potency of opioids is not an issue. Unwanted side effects are equivalent. An opioid is most likely indicated for a short duration, with 15 tablets being a reasonable amount for an injury of this type. The medication he obtained from the drug store was most likely an NSAID. (**Ref. 1,** p. 428; **Ref. 2,** p. 440; **Ref. 12,** p. 469)

655. E. All opioids cause dependence by stimulating mu, kappa, sigma, and delta receptors in the brain. These agents are effective in removing pain as suffering (emotion), but an individual may still identify the specific sensation. (**Ref. 1,** pp. 424, 428–429; **Ref. 2,** pp. 431–432, 437–439; **Ref. 4,** pp. 490–491; **Ref. 12,** p. 466)

656. C. Dextromethorphan is an antitussive with no addiction liability. Cough should not be managed with the agents that cause dependence or have the potential to cause dependence. Naloxone is an antagonist of morphine. (**Ref. 1,** p. 429; **Ref. 2,** pp. 446, 449; **Ref. 4,** pp. 503–504; **Ref. 12,** p. 474)

657. A. The use of an opioid compound is not indicated at this point. This is the mu receptor pathway. He is not in a chronic pain syndrome but such a syndrome may be prevented from developing by giving an NSAID. Acetaminophen, which has no anti-inflammatory action, should not be used. It would be appropriate to determine if phlebitis is present. (**Ref. 1,** pp. 494, 500; **Ref. 2,** p. 435; **Ref. 4,** pp. 501–502, 641; **Ref. 12,** pp. 536–537, 551)

658. B. Diphenoxylate is a meperidine derivative that is sold in a combination with atropine as Lomotil. It is a good choice for diarrhea. Opioids are not appropriate compounds. NSAIDs and acetaminophen are ineffective. Loperamide, another meperidine derivative, is widely and effectively used for diarrhea and is now available in a nonprescription strength. (**Ref. 1,** pp. 433, 894; **Ref. 2,** p. 445; **Ref. 4,** p. 507; **Ref. 12,** pp. 473–474)

659. B. Lomustine is used primarily in the treatment of brain tumors. In patients with one or more positive lymph nodes, CAF and CMF are most commonly given following surgery. Progestins, such as megestrol acetate, have been shown to be less effective than the antiestrogens. Taxol is usually reserved for refractory cases or tumors resistant to other agents. (**Ref. 2,** pp. 755, 695; **Ref. 8,** pp. 1302–1305; **Ref. 11,** pp. 284–288; **Ref. 12,** pp. 849–850)

660. D. Hypersensitivity reactions occur frequently during the first 15 to 60 minutes of an infusion. They are believed to be mediated by the release of histamine. Prophylaxis with corticosteroids, diphenhydramine, and cimetidine has significantly reduced the occurrence of such reactions. Symptoms include flushing rash, tachycardia, bronchospasm, hypotension, chest pain, and angioedema. (**Ref. 2,** pp. 694–695; **Ref. 8,** pp. 2355–2356; **Ref. 10,** pp. 673–674)

661. E. Tamoxifen has proven to be useful in the treatment of breast cancer, and it is also being used in the treatment of progesterone-resistant endometrial cancer. Tamoxifen acts as a competitive partial agonist-inhibitor of estrogen. It is particularly advantageous in that side effects are mild and do not include bone marrow suppression. (**Ref. 2,** pp. 696–697; **Ref. 4,** pp. 1256–1257; **Ref. 8,** pp. 1308–1309, 1317–1318; **Ref. 10,** pp. 689–692; **Ref. 11,** pp. 184–185; **Ref. 12,** p. 841)

662. B. Dimenhydrinate, while effective against motion-related nausea and vomiting, has little or no action against chemotherapy-induced nausea and vomiting. Prochlorperazine, dexamethasone, and lorazepam are all first-line agents in the treatment of chemotherapy-induced nausea and vomiting. The serotonin receptor antagonists ondansetron and granisetron are often reserved for highly emetic regimens or for patients refractory to other agents. (**Ref. 2,** pp. 830–837; **Ref. 4,** pp. 926–929; **Ref. 8,** pp. 2345–2346; **Ref. 11,** p. 431; **Ref. 12,** p. 954)

663. B. Vitamin D is used in the treatment of hypocalcemia. Initial treatment of hypercalcemia involves hydration and diuresis with a loop diuretic. If more prolonged treatment is needed, the following agents are used in order of preference: bisphosphonates, calcitonin, gallium nitrate, plicamycin, phosphate, and glucocorticoids. (**Ref. 2,** pp. 793–794; **Ref. 4,** pp. 1500–1501; **Ref. 12,** pp. 661–663)

664. D. The edema associated with pregnancy is probably due to the mineralocorticoid effect of estrogens. Current approaches lead away from drug use unless necessary. It may be uncomfortable, but most women tolerate the swelling fairly well. (**Ref. 2,** p. 220)

665. C. It is well recognized that drugs may cause problems at any stage of pregnancy and may pose problems during labor and delivery. Even conception may be adversely affected by drug use.

However, most birth defects occur during the first trimester, and pharmacologic agents should be avoided then. **(Ref. 1, p. 854; Ref. 2, p. 77; Ref. 12, pp. 913–914)**

666. **A.** The FDA does provide assigned risk categories; they are:

A—well-controlled studies show no apparent risk to humans
B—animal studies show no risk but no adequate studies in women
C—animal studies show risk, no adequate human studies
D—there is positive evidence of human risk based on adverse report data, but benefits may warrant the risk
X—positive data exists, and risks outweigh benefits

(Ref. 5, pp. 43–44; Ref. 6, p. x)

667. **E.** Oxytocin would be used to induce labor. The other agents can all be used to prevent premature labor. **(Ref. 1, pp. 121, 525; Ref. 2, pp. 729, 516; Ref. 4, pp. 949–950; Ref. 12, pp. 573–574)**

668. **D.** Change in diet and weight loss is the first step in the treatment of hyperlipidemia. Diet therapy and weight loss are usually tried for a minimum of 6 months before drug treatment is initiated. **(Ref. 1, pp. 482–483; Ref. 2, pp. 201–202; Ref. 12, p. 528)**

669. **C.** Niacin works to lower both plasma triglyceride and cholesterol levels. Niacin decreases cholesterol by inhibiting VLDL secretion, in turn decreasing production of LDL. Increased clearance of VLDL via the lipoprotein lipase pathway contributes to the triglyceride-lowering effects of niacin. **(Ref. 1, p. 483; Ref. 2, pp. 204–205; Ref. 12, p. 529)**

670. **A.** Most patients experience a prostaglandin-mediated cutaneous vasodilation with each dose upon the initiation of therapy or when the dose is increased. This side-effect can be blunted by prophylactic use of aspirin one-half hour prior to the niacin dose. Eventually, tachyphylaxis to this effect develops, and aspirin is no longer necessary. **(Ref. 1, p. 484; Ref. 2, p. 205; Ref. 12, p. 529)**

671. **A.** Decongestants are used in the treatment of sinus congestion. Antihistamines, H_1 antagonists, have all of the following actions: sedation, antiemetic and antinausea effects, antiparkinsonian

actions, anticholinergic effects, adrenoreceptor-blocking actions, serotonin-blocking actions, and local anesthetic effects. Each agent has differing degrees of each of these properties. (**Ref. 2, p. 818; Ref. 4, pp. 583–584; Ref. 12, pp. 257–258)**

672. **B.** Clemastine is an ethanolamine derivative with little or no sedative effects. It has greater anticholinergic effects than some of the other antihistamines. It is available orally both as a tablet and a liquid. (**Ref. 6, p. 306; Ref. 10, pp. 15–16)**

673. **D.** Severe cardiac arrhythmias have occurred in patients taking a combination of either terfenadine or astemizole and ketoconazole, itraconazole, or erythromycin. It is believed that the latter three drugs inhibit the metabolism of the antihistamines, resulting in increased blood concentrations. (**Ref. 2, p. 819; Ref. 12, p. 259)**

674. **C.** Cromolyn acts by reducing degranulation of mast cells triggered by IgE. Cromolyn is used in the prophylactic treatment of asthma, and must be used consistently on a daily basis in order to be effective. (**Ref. 2, pp. 821–822; Ref. 4, p. 630; Ref. 12, p. 255)**

675. **D.** While extensive investigation has been carried out, the statement that essentially nothing is known about its specific cause remains true. Drug therapy is often directed at choices A through C. (**Ref. 1, p. 139; Ref. 2, p. 229; Ref. 12, pp. 147–148)**

676. **B.** It is possible to lower blood pressure by therapeutic use of agents that influence the blood volume (kidneys), the cardiac output (heart), the central nervous system control of pressure (brain), or the contractile state of resistance or capacitance vessels (blood vessels). Other than altering the salt intake or nonpharmacological manipulation of pressure, the intestine does not play a role. (**Ref. 1, pp. 140–141; Ref. 2, pp. 229–230; Ref. 12, pp. 148–149)**

677. **A.** Cardiac glycosides would increase the inotropic activity of the heart and slow its rate. These agents are not antihypertensive agents even though they are used for congestive heart failure secondary to hypertension. All of the other choices are possible. (**Ref. 1, p. 141; Ref. 2, p. 230; Ref. 12, p. 149)**

678. E. Propranolol has its antihypertensive effect by an unknown mechanism. It depresses the rate and force of myocardial contraction by blocking β_1-receptors. This is thought to contribute to its effect. However, with continued treatment cardiac output returns to normal. β_1-receptor blockade inhibits renin production. (**Ref. 1,** pp. 149–150, 152; **Ref. 2,** pp. 239–240; **Ref. 12,** p. 157)

679. B. Ethanol is readily absorbed from the GI tract and metabolized in the liver. Toxicity in this case is due to alcohol, not acetaldehyde. It is true that men have more alcohol dehydrogenase in the stomach, thus they absorb less alcohol. (**Ref. 1,** pp. 320–321; **Ref. 2,** pp. 451–452; **Ref. 4,** p. 375; **Ref. 12,** pp. 350–351)

680. C. Ethanol is metabolized to CO_2 and water. Orientals have reduced acetaldehyde dehydrogenase, and consequently experience facial flushing, vasodilation, and tachycardia similar to a disulfiram reaction. This is a genetic deficiency. (**Ref. 2,** p. 452; **Ref. 4,** p. 375)

681. B. Usually, acute ethanol intoxication is not treated other than by supportive measures to maintain respiratory and cardiovascular function. The individual is allowed to sleep off the ethanol. It will be metabolized at a constant rate. Disulfiram is contraindicated and so are analeptics. (**Ref. 1,** pp. 325–327; **Ref. 4,** pp. 376–379; **Ref. 12,** pp. 355–356)

682. E. A diuretic would most likely increase the elimination of ethanol and not be of concern. However, cephalosporins and metronidazole can cause a disulfiram reaction due to inhibition of aldehyde dehydrogenase. Acetaminophen and alcohol have the potential to cause hepatotoxicity. Propoxyphene and other analgesics or sedatives will potentiate the depressant effect of ethanol. (**Ref. 1,** pp. 324–325; **Ref. 2,** pp. 455–456; **Ref. 12,** p. 354)

683. C. Hyperthyroidism causes warm, moist skin and excessive sweating. (**Ref. 8,** p. 1370; **Ref. 12,** pp. 582–583)

684. A. Synthetic levothyroxine is stable, inexpensive, and since T_4 is converted to T_3 intracellularly, administration of T_4 results in production of both T_4 and T_3. Liothyronine is shorter acting and more cardiotoxic than levothyroxine. Desiccated thyroid has greater protein antigenicity and methimazole and propylthiouracil are antithyroid agents. (**Ref. 4,** p. 1371; **Ref. 12,** p. 582)

685. **E.** Symptoms of hypothyroidism include all of these plus pale, cool skin, drooping eyelids, bradycardia, and infertility. (**Ref. 4,** p. 1371; **Ref. 12,** pp. 582–583)

686. **E.** Unneutralized $NaHCO_3$ is completely absorbed, and can cause transient metabolic alkalosis. If the pH of the stomach consistently stays above 5.5, the amount of acid secretion caused by a meal can be doubled. Bicarbonate neutralized in the stomach produces CO_2, causing abdominal distention, belching, and flatulence. Antacids given 1/2 to 1 hour after meals neutralize gastric acid for 2 hours. (**Ref. 4,** pp. 905–907; **Ref. 12,** p. 64)

687. **D.** Metoclopramide has little effect on gastric secretion. Taken before meals and at bedtime, it stimulates motility of the upper GI tract and decreases gastric emptying time. (**Ref. 4,** p. 928, **Ref. 12,** p. 953)

688. **B.** Calcium and magnesium carbonate both produce effects similar to those of sodium bicarbonate. Mg^{2+} salts cause diarrhea, while Al^{3+} salts yield constipation. Thiazides cause Ca^{2+} retention and the use of Al^{3+} to decrease PO_4 absorption in uremia is dangerous. (**Ref. 4,** pp. 985–986; **Ref. 12,** pp. 949–950)

689. **D.** Metoclopramide decreases gastric emptying time and enhances the motility of smooth muscle from the esophagus through the proximal small intestine. Large doses of $NaHCO_3$ and the ensuing belching can exacerbate gastroesophageal reflux, and taking $NaHCO_3$ with milk or cream can lead to the milk-alkali syndrome. (**Ref. 4,** pp. 905–907, 927; **Ref. 12,** p. 953)

690. **E.** While adverse effects with H_2-blocking drugs are relatively infrequent (usually less than 5%), headache, myalgia, dizziness, and nausea do occur. Ranitidine renders the stomach hypochlorhydric, favoring the formation of bezoars and microorganisms. Ranitidine does not cause tinnitus. (**Ref. 4,** pp. 900–901; **Ref. 12,** p. 951)

691. **E.** Agents that increase vagal tone suppress AV conduction and protect the ventricle. Compounds that decrease dV/dt in phase 4,

increase the refractory period, or increase resting membrane potential (making it more negative) would decrease arrhythmia production. (Ref. 1, pp. 194–195; Ref. 2, pp. 277–282; Ref. 4, pp. 841–845; Ref. 12, pp. 211–214; Ref. 13, pp. 155–158)

692. **A.** It is not unusual to have arrhythmia in individuals who are not well rested and who drink caffeine-containing beverages. Arrhythmias are always a sign of concern, but before instituting antiarrhythmic therapy, a careful analysis is needed. Reversible arrhythmias due to factors that can be changed do not require antiarrhythmic therapy. (Ref. 1, p. 190; Ref. 2, p. 311; Ref. 12, p. 205; Ref. 13, pp. 159–160)

693. **B.** While some of these agents might be appropriate, disopyramide would not be used. This is because of its anticholinergic effect, which would lead to urinary retention, especially in males with prostate problems. (Ref. 1, p. 201; Ref. 2, p. 290; Ref. 4, p. 857; Ref. 12, p. 218; Ref. 13, pp. 161, 169)

694. **D.** The antiarrhythmic agents are classified as I (sodium channel blockers), II (β-adrenergic blockers), III (agents that prolong action-potential duration), IV (calcium channel blockers), and others. In this last category is digitalis, which increases vagal tone. (Ref. 1, pp. 197–198; Ref. 2, pp. 283–284; Ref. 4, p. 847; Ref. 12, p. 214; Ref. 13, p. 163)

695. **D.** Arrhythmias must be carefully analyzed. Some are not candidates for drug therapy. When instituting drug therapy, it should be recognized that these drugs are toxic and that they may cause arrhythmias. (Ref. 2, p. 311; Ref. 12, pp. 205, 225–227)

696. **B.** Calcium channel blockers or β-adrenergic blockers are often the first choice for acute atrial fibrillation or flutter. (Ref. 1, p. 207; Ref. 2, p. 308; Ref. 4, p. 869; Ref. 12, pp. 223–224; Ref. 13, p. 167)

697. **E.** All are adverse effects of trimethoprim-sulfamethoxazole, but the most troublesome for Ms Spacey in the interaction with sodium warfarin, which has probably brought on GI bleeding, accounting for the blood she has spit up. (Ref. 1, pp. 469–470; Ref. 6, pp. 238, 2523–2524, 2715; Ref. 12, p. 514)

698. E. Antidiabetic agents displace protein-bound anticoagulants. Aspirin increases anticoagulant activity by its effect on platelet aggregation, and third-generation cephalosporins eliminate Vitamin K–producing bacteria from the GI tract. Barbiturates cause hepatic enzyme induction, which decreases anticoagulant activity. (**Ref. 1**, pp. 469–470; **Ref. 6**, pp. 235–239; **Ref. 12**, p. 514)

699. E. Antacids and sucralfate decrease anticoagulant activity by decreasing absorption from the GI tract while cimetidine brings about an increase in anticoagulant activity by inhibition of their hepatic enzymatic metabolism. (**Ref. 1**, p. 470; **Ref. 6**, pp. 235–239; **Ref. 12**, p. 514)

700. E. Each of the other listed conditions is an accepted indication for anticoagulant therapy. Anticoagulant therapy can be risky in patients with ulceration or other lesions of the GI tract. (**Ref. 1**, p. 469; **Ref. 6**, pp. 230, 232–233; **Ref. 12**, pp. 512–513)

References

1. Katzung BG: *Basic and Clinical Pharmacology,* 5th ed. Norwalk, CT, San Mateo, CA, Appleton & Lange, 1992.

2. Craig CR, Stitzel RE: *Modern Pharmacology,* 4th ed. Boston, Little, Brown, 1994.

3. Clark WG, Brater DC, Johnson AR: *Goth's Medical Pharmacology,* 13th ed. Boston, Mosby Year Book, 1992.

4. Gilman AG, Rall TW, Nies AS, et al: *The Pharmacological Basis of Therapeutics,* 8th ed. New York, Pergamon Press, 1990.

5. *Drug Evaluations Annual 1994.* Chicago, American Medical Association, 1994.

6. *USP DI Volume 1, Drug Information for the Health Care Professional.* Rockville, MD, United States Pharmacopeial Convention, Inc., 1994.

7. Pratt WB, Taylor P: *Principles of Drug Action,* 3rd ed. New York, Churchill Livingstone, 1990.

8. DeVita VT Jr, Hellman S, Rosenberg SA: *Cancer: Principles & Practice of Oncology,* 4th ed. Philadelphia, PA, JB Lippincott, 1993.

9. *Physicians Desk Reference,* 48th ed. Oradell, NJ, Medical Economics Co., 1994.

10. *American Hospital Formulary Service: Drug Information 94.* Bethesda, MD, American Society of Hospital Pharmacists, Inc., 1994.

11. Fisher DS, Knobf MT: *The Cancer Chemotherapy Handbook.* Chicago, Yearbook Medical Publishers, 1989.

12. Katzung BG: *Basic & Clinical Pharmacology,* 6th ed. Norwalk, CT, San Mateo, CA, Appleton & Lange, 1995.

13. Melmon KL, Morrelli HF, Hoffman BB, Nierenberg DW: *Melmon & Morrelli's Clinical Pharmacology,* 3rd ed. New York, McGraw-Hill, 1992.